An Introduction to Qualitative Methods for Health Professionals

MADELEINE GANTLEY, GEOFFREY HARDING,
SATINDER KUMAR, JO TISSIER

Published by
The Royal College of General Practitioners
1999

The Royal College of General Practitioners
was founded in 1952 with this object:

"To encourage, foster and maintain the highest possible standards in general practice and for that purpose to take or join with others in taking steps consistent with the charitable nature of that object
which may assist towards the same."

Among its responsibilities under its Royal Charter
the College is entitled to:

"Encourage the publication by general medical practitioners of research into medical or scientific subjects with a view to the improvement of general medical practice in any field and to undertake or assist
others in undertaking such research.

Diffuse information on all matters affecting general practice and establish, print, publish, issue and cir-
culate such papers, journals, magazines, books, periodicals, and publications and hold such meetings,
conferences, seminars and instructional courses as may assist the object of the College."

First impression 1999

Published by the Royal College of General Practitioners
14 Princes Gate
Hyde Park
London, SW7 1PU

Printed and bound by BSC Print Ltd, Wimbledon

ISBN 0 85084 246 8

CONTENTS

The qualitative researcher has been compared to Manuel, the waiter:

'permanently harassed by those in authority and failing to communicate urgent news because he cannot speak their language'.

(Dingwall, 1992)

· 1 ·

WHAT IS QUALITATIVE RESEARCH?

DEFINITIONS

There is enormous debate over the term qualitative research. We use it here to refer to research using qualitative methods of data collection, and qualitative methods of data analysis. This does not include what is sometimes termed 'converting opinions into numbers' i.e. collecting data on, for instance, patient satisfaction, attributing numerical values to individual views and subjecting them to quantitative analysis.

One of the most explicit definitions of qualitative research is drawn from the *Handbook of Qualitative Research*:

'Qualitative research is multi-method in focus, involving an interpretive, naturalistic approach to its subject matter. This means that qualitative researchers study things in their natural settings, attempting to make sense of, or interpret, phenomena in terms of the meanings people bring to them.' (Denzin and Lincoln, 1994.)

This definition emphasises both the need for multiple methods of data collection, and an interpretive, naturalistic approach. Data collection takes place in as natural a way as possible: in informants' own homes, at times of their choosing, and using language and priorities reflecting informants' own beliefs and experiences. The researcher is an integral part of the research process, and is expected to reflect on his or her own influence on data collection. This is in stark contrast to the controlled, artificial environment of experimental research, where the researcher is an apparently neutral observer, distant from the research setting.

The focus on interpretation and meaning has a number of implications, particularly for health professionals:

1. Interpretive analysis concentrates on understanding the views of research participants; it makes explicit the distinction between respondents' views and the researcher's interpretations;
2. Interpretive analysis accepts that there are different coexisting interpretations of any phenomenon, e.g. a sore throat, and attaches equal importance to each interpretation;
3. The recognition of multiple meanings challenges one of the basic tenets of western biomedicine and evidence-based medicine, that of **positivism**.

> ## EXERCISE 1
>
> Read journal Articles 1 to 3 in the workbook: Why is an understanding of postmodernism, positivism and 'anti-positivism' important for health researchers undertaking qualitative research?
>
> *Your answer should reflect the following points:*
> - ***positivism** has been the dominant mode of explanation for the last 400 years or so*
> - *qualitative research draws on different paradigms, sometimes characterised as '**anti-positivism**'*
> - *the majority of health-related research uses a linear **hypothetico-deductive** process, while qualitative research uses an **iterative-inductive** process.*

WHAT SORT OF QUESTIONS CAN QUALITATIVE RESEARCH ADDRESS?

When choosing specific research methods, the key consideration is the nature of the research question. Qualitative research is essentially '**exploratory**', setting out to describe, understand and explain a particular phenomenon. It may address 'what?', 'why?' and 'how?' but not 'how many?' or 'how frequently?'.

In health services research, qualitative studies may stand alone or may be involved at different stages of the research process in conjunction with quantitative studies. Some of the most frequent qualitative research questions address processes and beliefs, for example:

1. **Process**, i.e. how an outcome is reached or why a particular course of action is followed, e.g. 'Recognising meningococcal disease in primary care: qualitative study of how general practitioners process clinical and contextual information' (Granier et al, 1998).
2. **Ideas or beliefs**, e.g. 'Health beliefs and folk models of diabetes in British Bangladeshis: a qualitative study.' (Greenhalgh T, Helman C and Chowdhury AM, 1998).

Qualitative research may also involve building theoretical models:

3. **Hypothesis generation** or '**grounded theory**' (see *Grounded Theory*, p17: when the categories or outcomes of the research cannot be determined before data collection is undertaken, the research may lead to hypothesis generation or grounded theory rather than hypothesis testing, e.g. 'What worries parents when their pre-school children are acutely ill, and why: a qualitative study' (Kai, 1996).

All of the examples cited here are drawn from medical journals, and are designed to contribute to an understanding of topics which are specifically relevant to primary care and general practice.

Journals such as the *British Medical Journal*, the *British Journal of General Practice*, *Family Practice*, *Quality in Health Care*, and the *Scandinavian Journal of Primary Health Care* publish papers using qualitative methodology. Other examples of qualitative research, often grounded explicitly within the disciplines of sociology, anthropology or psychology, may be found in journals such as *Sociology of Health and Illness*, *Social Science and Medicine*, or *Qualitative Health Research*.

EXERCISE 2

Read Articles 4 to 6 (as cited above).
What are the strengths and weaknesses of qualitative research?
What are the implications for health professionals undertaking qualitative research?

Your answers should include the following
Strengths:
- *qualitative research allows the researcher to explore the meanings that respondents attach to particular experiences*
- *qualitative research is open ended: respondents' own priorities are allowed to lead the data collection*
- *small samples allow rich (i.e. detailed) data to be obtained*
- *the data is context rich, the researcher is able to use complementary data sources*
- *multiple methods may be used, such as interviews, focus groups and observation*
- *the validity of the data is established through confirmation with research participants.*

Weaknesses:
- *data is context specific, and is not intended to be generalisable to other contexts*
- *the researcher has an impact on the data collected*
- *small samples are used.*

Implications for health professionals:
- *Health professionals' own identity and status will affect the nature of the data collected*
- *Health professionals may be working, consciously or unconsciously, with their own professional beliefs and priorities*
- *The positivist orientation of the majority of health services research may limit the analytical potential of the research.*

· 2 ·

METHODS OF DATA COLLECTION

As our original definition of qualitative research suggests, there are a variety of ways to collect qualitative research data. Each has strengths and weaknesses which should be considered before beginning.

Read Articles 7 to 9 before looking at the following practical exercises.

EXERCISE 3

Interviews

Imagine you (a GP) are about to interview someone (for instance, a younger colleague) about their working day. How would you proceed?

- think about the purpose of the research
- think about the type of topics you would like to address
- read the existing research in this area
- prepare a topic guide
- develop the topic guide into potential questions
- draft open and closed questions
- prepare prompts and probes.

Take time to plan an interview, and conduct it (ideally with a sympathetic colleague):

- where will the interview take place?
- how long will it last?
- how will you describe the research to your informant?
- what ethical issues are involved?
- is confidentiality an issue? How will this affect the data?
- how will data be recorded and analysed?
- how will you keep the interviewee 'on track'?
- what kind of notes will you take during the interview?

Take time to reflect:

- how does interviewing differ from a consultation?
- what type of questions did you ask?
- what does this say about your own interests and priorities?
- how did the data relate to the existing literature?
- discuss your interpretations with a colleague from a different discipline: if they differ, why do they?

Your answers should include the following points
- *a consultation is time limited, and has a focus on identifying and meeting the patient's needs and the health professional's responsibilities*
- *a research interview is essentially open ended and exploratory, with the respondent encouraged to influence the course of the discussion*
- *your own questions may reflect your own priorities rather than those of your respondent: consider how a question on, say, free time may be interpreted by a younger colleague*
- *your own questions may affect the responses.*

EXERCISE 4

Focus Groups

Imagine you (a practice nurse) have decided to run focus groups on how your multi-professional colleagues see the future of primary care nursing. How would you proceed?

- think about the purpose of the research
- think about the type of topics you would like to address
- read existing literature or policy documents
- prepare a topic guide
- develop the topic guide into potential questions
- use open and closed questions
- prepare prompts and probes.

Take time to plan a small focus group, and to conduct it (perhaps with other nurse researchers). Bear in mind the following points:

- where will the focus group take place?
- how will the seating be arranged?
- how long will it last?
- how will you describe the research to group members?
- what ethical issues are involved?
- is confidentiality an issue? How will this affect the data?
- how will data be recorded and analysed?
- what kind of notes will you take during the interview?
- will an observer/facilitator be available to take additional notes?
- how will you encourage contributions from 'quiet' participants?
- how will you discourage the 'dominant' group member?

Provide a simple diagram showing the seating arrangements, and ask the observer to 'map' group interactions by drawing a pencil line between participants, or between facilitator and participant, to show each interaction. The aim of the focus group is to encourage group members to talk to each other, and this simple mapping exercise shows how much this actually happens (Figure 1):

In Figure 1, it is possible to identify the facilitator because comments or questions have originated largely from one point in the circle. The arrows between participants reveal that some lateral dialogue has been prompted, but there is a participant who has not spoken to any other members of the group.

Take time to reflect:

- how has running a focus group differed from interviewing?

Figure 1: Focus Group – sharing the interaction between members

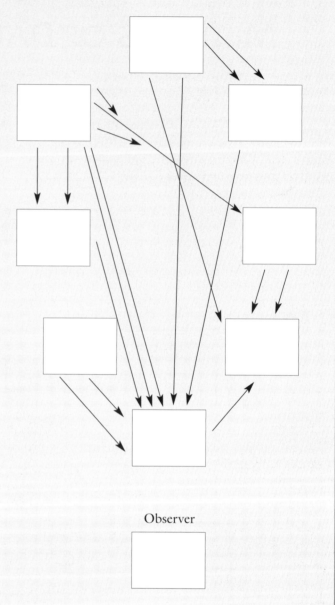

Observer

- what implications are there for the nature of the data collected?
- are there implications for the research process?
- discuss your interpretations with a colleague from a different discipline. Do they differ? If so, why?

Your answers should include the following points:

- *focus groups provide the opportunity to collect a range of data relatively quickly*
- *however, people may not turn up*
- *it may be difficult to guide the discussion in order to gather relevant data*
- *dominant group members may inhibit others*
- *recording and transcribing are technically difficult.*

EXERCISE 5

Observation

Imagine you (a social scientist) are about to conduct some interviews with a variety of members of a practice team. Why would a short period of observation be helpful?

- observation provides an insight into the whole research setting
- people are seen in their 'natural' setting
- process and interactions may be observed
- it involves observing what people do, rather than what they say they do.

Take time to observe a setting with which you are familiar (e.g. a general practice), and imagine being an unfamiliar observer. This is a process that anthropologists term 'making the familiar strange', and is designed to encourage observers to recognise familiar 'routine accomplishments', which are essential elements of qualitative research. The following are features worth observing:

- what kind of magazines or leaflets are available?
- in what languages are leaflets available?
- how GPs and receptionists address each other? First names or titles?
- how the practice manager and GPs address each other?
- how reception staff manage when surgeries run late?
- who makes the coffee?
- what kind of provision is there for young children e.g. toys, etc?
- what security measures are in place?
- how reception staff deal with patients, in person and on the phone?

You might expect to learn the following:

- *that the practice has a commitment to providing health education information, provision for speakers of languages other than English, and provision for young children in the waiting room*
- *that the practice does not make these provisions*
- *the apparent nature of inter-professional relationships (e.g. tense, informal, unequal, joking, good tempered, bad tempered)*
- *coping strategies adopted by reception staff (e.g. talking informally to patients when the GP is delayed).*

EXERCISE 6

Data Collection

Take time to reflect: How has using observational data informed the data collection process?

Your answer should include the following points:
- *observation may sensitise the observer to questions for further research, e.g. inter-professional relations, or a commitment to health education*
- *observation allows an understanding of the management of space and time, both highly ordered in a general practice surgery*

EXERCISE 7

Comparing Methods of Data Collection

Now try to summarise the advantages and disadvantages of each of these methods in the Tables 1 to 3:

Table 1
Interviews

Advantages	Disadvantages

Table 2
Focus Groups

Advantages	Disadvantages

Table 3
Observation

Advantages	Disadvantages

Check your answers by reading Article 10.

Complementary data collection methods such as observation followed by interviews, or focus groups followed by interviews, or interviews followed by focus groups, are often used to maximise the rigour of the research.

EXERCISE 8

Tourism and Romanticism
Read Article 11.

Explain the potential dangers of tourism and romanticism.

Your answer should include the following points:
- 'Tourism'
Starting research without a hypothesis, the tourist/researcher seeks new and different activities; the tourist/researcher may fail to recognise similarities between their own and 'other' cultures

- 'Romanticism'
The researcher sets out to record and explain the experiences of a usually disadvantaged group; this approach may neglect how this experience is shaped by the cultural influences on both individuals and social groups.
What strategies does Silverman suggest to help researchers avoid tourism and romanticism?

· 3 ·
SAMPLING

Selecting a sampling strategy for qualitative research is crucial. Again there are distinct differences from quantitative approaches.

While quantitative research relies on larger random probability samples chosen for representativeness and the potential for generalisation, qualitative research relies on sampling strategies which allow the researcher to claim either that a full range of views or experiences have been investigated, or that the data have provided the grounds for theoretical development.

For an overview of sampling strategies, see Patton MQ (1990). Chapter 5 identifies 16 types of sampling, all grouped under the general heading of 'purposeful'.

EXERCISE 9

Sampling

Read Article 12.
The following are some of the most common sampling strategies adopted. What do you understand by these terms? Fill in Table 4:

Table 4

Intensity sampling:

_____

Maximum variation sampling:

_____

Typical case sampling:

_____

Snowball or **chain** sampling:

_____

Confirming and **disconfirming** cases:

_____

It is common for several different sampling strategies to be adopted within one study. This has the advantage of allowing **triangulation** of data, an important feature in ensuring the validity of the analysis (see Chapter 5).

· 4 ·

DATA ANALYSIS

There are two essential processes in data analysis, the first is 'data management', i.e. recording, transcribing tapes, managing observational and field notes, and the second is the work of the analysis.

DATA MANAGEMENT

Interviews, focus groups and observation produce massive amounts of data, either paper transcripts or extensive computer files. There are a number of computer programs available for the analysis of qualitative data. For a review, see Tesch R (1991). Below are some pointers to help you organise your data:

- set up computer or paper files with a chronological record of all data collection episodes
- under each data set file notes taken at the time of the interview, and the transcript
- include any other relevant demographic data on each interviewee
- keep a record of any changes or additions made to the interview guide
- keep a record of any analytical insights which led to these changes
- ensure that all data is anonymised, and that guarantees of confidentiality are respected through secure storage and careful record keeping.

As mentioned earlier, qualitative data analysis is an **iterative process**, starting at the very earliest stages of the data collection.

> **EXERCISE 10**
>
> Read Article 13.
> What do you understand by **analytic induction**?
> What do you understand by **grounded theory**?
> Bryman and Burgess (1994) identify the processes of **generation of concepts** and building of **typologies** and **taxonomies**'. What do you understand by each of these?
>
> *Your answers should reflect your understanding of the material after working through the exercise. Further information on the key areas is included in the section on approaches to analysis.*

APPROACHES TO ANALYSIS

There are a range of different ways of analysing qualitative data, and here we summarise four of them. Each of these approaches was the subject of a workshop at the one-day class for which this handbook was prepared, and each of the workshop leaders has contributed the relevant section. The methods have been chosen for their relevance to primary care research.

> *Collecting all your data and then turning hopefully to a qualitative researcher saying 'what do I do now?' is the wrong way to do qualitative research, and will not make you friends.*

1 A BEGINNER'S GUIDE TO DEVELOPING A THEMATIC ANALYSIS

Madeleine Gantley

Qualitative data analysis is complex, and reducing it a series of steps risks massive over-simplification. However, the basic steps are set out here:

Reflection

Reflect on every period of data collection, and immediately record ideas of potential analytical points. Read data thoroughly as soon as transcripts are available, and identify issues (low level topics), categories (groups of issues) and analytical themes (theoretical perspectives linking the categories): see Table 5. Note that different authors use different terms to identify this process but the essential principle – that of identifying increasing levels of abstraction – remains throughout.

Developing an analytical framework
Indexing

Develop a system of indexing all data, so that each mention of a particular issue is easily identifiable and retrievable. Review the index to ensure that it is comprehensive, and does not omit any of the data (or, if you do have data that are beyond the scope of the analysis being undertaken, note this in the methodological description).

Method review

Review sampling, topic guide and data collection methods in order to maximise opportunities to develop and challenge the emergent analysis, and to review the analysis with future interviewees. Continue collecting data, and reviewing the analytical framework in the light of each data set, and relevant literature.

Framework
Apply the analytical **framework** to all the data collected, seeking out inconsistencies and questions. Continue collecting data until **saturation** is reached, i.e. until no new data are generated by interviewees. In practice this may be limited by the time or budget available.

The following data is a short anonymised extract from one of a series of interviews conducted after completion of the LIZEI (London Implementation Zone, Educational Incentives) scheme.

From Table 5 it is possible to identify the following issues, categories and themes:

Table 5

Interview (LIZEI Scheme)

(I)=Interviewer; (GP)=GP respondent

(I): And how did you decide what you wanted to do?

(GP): There were certain things that we were doing, one was fundholding, we're going into this, and we had the meetings, loads and loads of meetings...

(I): Did you have a plan of what education you wanted to do?

(GP): No, it was basically the courses as, and when they came, we chose which we wanted to do and which we didn't want to do.

(I): What has the funding enabled you to do?

(GP): To do the courses and get paid at the same time.

Issues:
- decision making
- fundholding
- meetings
- courses as, and when, they came
- getting paid.

Categories:
- actual activities, e.g. fundholding
- attending courses
- importance of funding.

Analytical themes:
- Essentially *reactive* strategy, claiming money for activities that would have been undertaken anyway, undertaking courses reactively rather than proactively
- *Accumulating* small amounts of money rather than claiming one larger sum; this was in contrast to other individual or groups of GPs who put in bids for significant programmes of activity that they had intended to undertake regardless of the availability of LIZEI funding
- The GP as independent contractor, concerned at the financial status of the practice, and following the priorities of **managerialism** (a term used in the social sciences to describe the dominance of the managerial agenda).

Bear in mind that the analytical themes are influenced by both the demands of the research, and the disciplinary context of the research and the researcher. This evaluative research for the Department of General Practice and Primary Care at Queen Mary and Westfield College, and for the wider educational providers in primary care in London, was concerned to look at how people had made use of LIZEI money. It looked at if and how they planned their educational activities, and the implications for the future.

Conclusion
By comparing data, it became clear that some claimants were proactive and some reactive in their educational activities. Some were accumulating a series of small sums of money while others were 'big bidders', and for some the provision of earmarked funding had been central to their decisions in relation to educational activities. Read the extract critically, from the point of view of the interviewer. Note the intitial use of an open question, followed by increasingly closed questions designed to focus the respondent on the research agenda.

2 CHARTING

Jo Tissier

Charting is one of five stages involved in an analytic approach called **Framework**, which was developed by an independent social research institute, Social and Community Planning Research. Framework can be used for qualitative data analysis for applied research. It is systematic and disciplined but it also relies on the creativity of the analyst to create meaning and connections. The five stages involved are:

- familiarisation
- identification of a thematic framework
- indexing
- charting
- mapping and interpretation.

Although the five steps appear to be separate, they are all highly interconnected. A brief overview of each stage is given below.

Familiarisation
Essentially this is the initial stage during which the analyst becomes familiar with the data through reading and re-reading transcripts. Research notes are made listing key ideas and themes.

Identifying a thematic framework

Once the data have been reviewed, the analyst returns to the research notes, and attempts to identify key issues, concepts and themes. This provides a framework or index within which the material can be sorted. The development of this index will draw on the research aims, as well as issues raised by the respondents themselves. The index is applied to a few transcripts and the categories are refined. The index may go through many draft stages and the process can be time-consuming.

Indexing

This is the process whereby the index is systematically applied to the data. All the data is read and annotated according to the index.

Charting

Charting refers to the process whereby data is taken from the transcripts and reassembled according to the appropriate thematic reference. Charts are devised with headings and subheadings drawn from the thematic framework, from the research questions or according to how the research will be presented. In the case of one study, evaluating GPs' educational opportunities, I drew up charts for each group of respondents: e.g. academic trainee GPs and GPs in full-time practice. Transcripts were coded with the appropriate index references and a summary of each respondent's views entered on the chart.

Table 6 shows an example of this chart illustrating the kind of entries recorded together with the page referencing system. I use large sheets of paper and different coloured pens to illustrate whether the entry is a direct quote or a summary of a respondent's view. In this extract, italics are used to show direct quotes. The use of charts affords several interpretations of data: review of individual rows allows the summary of one respondent's responses, and review of individual columns allows the contrasting of different respondents' experiences.

Mapping and interpretation

When all the data have been sifted and charted, the analyst brings together its key characteristics, and interprets the data set as a whole. This process will be guided by the original research questions and by themes that have arisen from the data.

Conclusion

Framework is just one approach for interpreting qualitative data. It documents each stage of the process of analysis and is a useful method in that it can give some structure to what may initially seem an unwieldy dataset.

Suggested reading

Ritchie J and Spencer L (1994) Qualitative data analysis for applied policy research. In Bryman A and Burgess R (eds) *Analysing Qualitative Data*. London, Routledge.

TABLE 6
Charting

London Academic Trainee	Activities before scheme	Experience as a GP in East London	Influence of LATs on career development	Contribution of scheme to general practice
Respondent 1	Just finished vocational training scheme. *'I felt I had to do it, because VTS did not prepare me fully as a GP because there is no research'* (p1)	No experience (p1) *'I live in East London and my future is in East London'* (p2)	Benefits: *'a tremendous gain'* (p3). Weak points: *'most of the time you are on your own'* (p3)	*'GPs need to take the lead on doing research in the community but lack the skills'* (p6)
Respondent 2	Parenthood. Seeking part-time work (p1)	Did vocational training scheme in East London (p1)	*'Brilliant stepping stone to know which aspect I want to do in the future, whether I want to go down the academic path or not'* (p4) Unsure about academic future (p4)	More satisfying than being a locum but less satisfying than being a principal (p4)

3 GROUNDED THEORY
Satinder Kumar

This section introduces **grounded theory**, summarises the analytical process, and reflects on the popularity of specific versions of grounded theory in general practice research.

Among the range of qualitative methods available, grounded theory is distinguished by its emphasis on method and its structured approach to data collection and analysis. This was the result of a conscious effort on the part of its co-founders, Glaser and Strauss, to redress criticisms of qualitative research as impressionistic and lacking structure and credibility (Glaser and Strauss, 1967).

Grounded theory
- provides an explicit and orderly guide for the collection and analysis of data
- provides explicit criteria on how grounded theory can be judged
- can generate hypotheses, substantive and, ultimately, formal theories
- makes claims for generalisability when a formal grounded theory is produced
- provides a potential to link to quantitative work e.g. through the discovery of hypotheses or the development of questionnaires.

Why grounded theory?
The aim of a grounded theory study is to discover or generate a theory/hypothesis that relates to a particular situation.

For example, I aimed – as a GP researcher – to generate hypotheses that related advances in medical genetics to the role of general practitioners as medical generalists. Specifically, I wanted to research how GP's perception of themselves, as generalists practising holistic medicine, would be re-shaped by new and highly specialised genetic knowledge that promoted a deterministic approach to clinical practice. Briefly, this involved studying how GPs acted and reacted to advances in genetics by collecting primarily interview data, then identifying, developing and interrelating categories from the data and finally developing theoretical propositions or hypotheses.

An overview of grounded theory data collection and analysis
Data collection usually involves 20 to 30 interviews with informants theoretically selected. Theoretical sampling is used to maximise the discovery of theory/hypotheses. Sampling, data collection and analysis are iterative i.e. data collection and analysis occur in tandem and both influence future sampling decisions. Data analysis is carried out by collecting data and comparing it to emerging categories, defined by Strauss and Corbin (1990) as **units of information** identified in the data. Data collection continues until categories reach **saturation**, i.e. until no more information explaining a category can be found.

Open coding
This is the first stage of the analytical process. A script is open coded by identifying primary or initial categories of information about the situation or phenomenon being studied. This is achieved by fragmenting the data, analysing sentences and phrases individually to label categories which in turn are described in more detail in terms of their **properties** or **dimensions**. At this stage, the researcher will need to reflect on the need to collect more data to explore the properties or dimensions as fully as possible, which will in turn determine who subsequent informants should be.

Axial coding
This is the next stage. Here the researcher reassembles the open coded data in new ways, often shown as a diagram, or analytical framework. This consists of core categories developed from the open coded data. The diagram often shows the links between core categories and factors that influence them. In addition, this stage involves identifying specific actions and/or interactions that result from the core category, as well as identifying the contexts that influence the core category.

Selective coding
The final stage is selective coding. Here the researcher identifies a 'story' and writes a narrative that integrates all the categories in the axial coding stage. It is during this phase that hypotheses may be presented. Finally, the researcher may relate the analysis to social, economic, political and historical factors that influence the analysis. This latter stage of analysis is not often seen in grounded theory work from primary care.

Constant comparative method
This approach to analysis is called the **constant comparative method** as it involves drawing information from the data collected and comparing it to emerging categories. The outcome of a grounded theory study is the production of a plausible relationship between concepts or groups of concepts. This may be presented in the form of a narrative statement, a visual picture, or a series of propositions or hypotheses.

Grounded theory and primary care researchers
Glaser and Strauss have each elaborated the theory they co-founded, individually, and in conjunction with others (e.g. Glaser 1978, 1992, Strauss 1987, and Strauss and Corbin 1990). However, while Strauss' work has focused on describing the method further, Glaser has developed more theoretical aspects.

Uses in biomedicine
The procedural emphasis in Strauss and Corbin's version of grounded theory may explain why it speaks so directly to researchers with a biomedical background.

Table 7
Representation of grounded theory analysis:

Extract from Interview 1	*Initial categories*	*Extract from Interview 5*	*Initial categories*
SK: When do you raise the issue of genetic risk?	Avoiding genetic risk	SK: When do you raise the issue of genetic risk?	GP Fatalism
	No effective intervention		Death sentence
GP: *I don't raise the issue- not for breast and ovarian cancer because there is nothing positive that can be done at present. Raising the issue would only make the patient and the family anxious.*	Awareness and anxiety	GP: *The problem with breast cancer – what can you do if you've got the gene? Is there any sense in giving a potential death sentence? If at the moment we can't alter the natural history then I can't see myself raising the issue*	Alter history
			No treatment/prevention.

Step 1: Open coding.
Open coding clarified questions to be asked in subsequent interviews e.g. Can you describe situations where you may be compelled to discuss genetic risk for breast cancer?

Step 2: Axial coding   *Step 3: Core Categories*

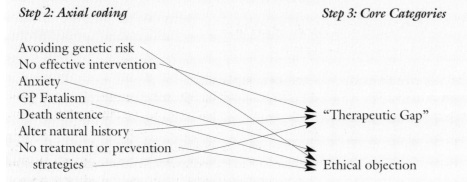

Avoiding genetic risk
No effective intervention
Anxiety
GP Fatalism
Death sentence
Alter natural history
No treatment or prevention
   strategies

"Therapeutic Gap"

Ethical objection

Step 4: Selective coding: "Identifying a story."

Ethical dilemmas associated with the therapeutic gap: "I don't raise the issue because there is nothing positive that can be done..."

GPs were reluctant to alert patients to genetic risk in the absence of effective screening technologies and therapies to reduce risk or prevent disease – in other words they identified a 'therapeutic gap' as an ethical dilemma. By raising the issue of genetic risk GPs thought they would create anxiety.

In practice these steps are not linear but iterative – sampling, data collection and analysis occurs simultaneously and so may all steps in analysis

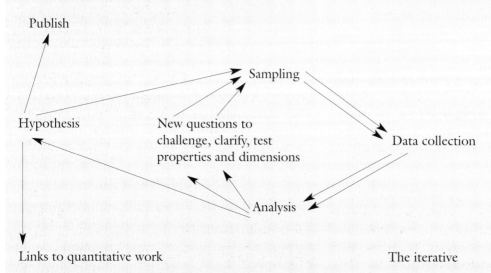

Publish

Sampling

Hypothesis

New questions to challenge, clarify, test properties and dimensions

Data collection

Analysis

Links to quantitative work   The iterative

For in biomedicine we find it more acceptable to conduct research within a strict framework. To produce a bona fide grounded theory, the researcher needs to observe strict procedures. This is in direct contrast to many other qualitative methods which see the focus on methodological procedure as a distraction from understanding and giving meaning to data (Janesick, 1994).

Conclusion

Research using grounded theory is a substantial undertaking in terms of time, hours of work and financial resources. In the context of biomedical research, it is not always feasible. Although other methods of qualitative data collection and analysis may be more feasible, authors often cite the use of 'grounded theory approach'; use of the term in research papers signals a commitment to certain procedural steps in sampling, data collection and analysis.

Suggested reading

Glaser B (1978) *Theoretical Sensitivity*. Mill Valley, CA, Sociological Press

Glaser B (1992) *Emergence vs. Forcing; Basics of Grounded Theory Analysis*. Mill Valley, CA, Sociological Press

Glaser B and Strauss A (1967) *The Discovery of Grounded Theory*. CA, Aldine

Janesick VJ (1994) The dance of qualitative research design. Metaphor, methodolatry, and meaning. In Denzin N and Lincoln Y (eds) *Handbook of Qualitative Research* CA, Sage

Strauss A (1987) *Qualitative Analysis for Social Scientists*. New York, Cambridge University Press

Strauss A and Corbin J (1990) *Basics of Qualitative Research*. London, Sage

4 NARRATIVE ANALYSIS
Geoffrey Harding

Narrative analysis offers a different way of approaching qualitative data analysis. Some issues in primary care research do not readily lend themselves to investigation by the popular method of focus groups because of their nature and characteristics.

A place for narrative analysis

For example, a person's experience of bereavement, or illicit drug use, may not be appropriate topics for focus groups because of the intrinsic sensitivity of these issues. In-depth interviews are a more appropriate methodological tool, but again, because of their nature, **charting** as a means of analysis may not be appropriate because it involves exploring emergent themes resulting from the disaggregation of transcripts.

In disaggregating narratives, it has been argued that the structure of people's responses becomes fractured and consequently potentially important aspects of these accounts – their sequence and structure – are lost.

Story as 'self'

In certain instances, for example, the experience of bereavement, the accounts can be very densely emotional, and 'fracturing' them to elicit themes may be argued to be an insensitive analytical approach in that it fails to recognise that they are coherent personal accounts. The telling of one's 'story' is not simply an account of a personal experience, it is also a way to fashion one's identity.

To take an example, in a study of consultations between a consultant paediatric cardiologist and parents of children with Down's syndrome, Baruch (1981) was able to show, using a narrative analysis, that parents used the consultation with a cardiologist to fashion their identity as 'good' parents.

Finding a structure

A central assumption of narrative analysis is that respondents, whether as interviewees in an in-depth interview, or in artificial settings e.g. patients in medical settings, impose order on their recounted experiences to make sense of these events and actions. The analyst's task is to explore how recounted events and experiences are put together by first identifying the story and then illuminating its structure. Clearly not all narration comprises of clearly identified 'stories', and some interpretation to find which narration contains analysable stories is required.

Narrative analysis differs from other qualitative analytical approaches in that the transcript requires to be structured in some detail. An example of such an annotated transcript follows:

TABLE 8
Transcript
(P)=parent (I)=interviewer

1. (P) Well the story really started with him going in for
2.   a minor op last year and the anaesthetist just er
3.   investigations discovered a murmur which she wasn't
4.   very happy about and referred us to a paediatrician
5.   after the op who agreed that it was an unusual sight
6.   and um
7.   murmurs are commonplace really
8. (I) um
9. (P) But on the sight and nature of it, it sort of wanted
10.   further investigation.

(Silverman, 1993)

Method

There are several means of analysing transcripts. A particularly useful starting point is to examine how narratives are organised. Identifying instances where the narration orientates the listener, where action is described, how the action is evaluated and how the action is resolved, may do this. As with all qualitative analyses, this can only be achieved through close and repeated listening to the taped recordings and methodical transcribing. By doing so, the aim is to interpret the narrator's strategy to construct the story in order for it to make sense.

Clearly there are a number of different interpretations to be made of any narrative, but, as Riessman (1990) observes, "The teller has, if not the final word, at least the first word on which interpretation depends." She continues:

"When I was analysing Cindy's long narrative, I was led into my sense of it by its organisation. She could have said what she had to say in several different ways. What did the form she chose signify? I claim that we can come close to seeing into her subjective experience – what life "means" to her at the moment of telling – through experiencing the tension in the structure of the narrative (the juxtaposition of the real and the wished for, the story and the dream")).

Conclusion

The relevance to primary care research of establishing how people construct their identities in such circumstances is in showing how people construct an image of themselves in certain circumstances. Knowing how people fashion their identities has implications for the ways in which people use primary care services.

Suggested reading

Baruch G (1981) Moral tales: parents' stories of encounters with the health professional. *Sociology of Health and Illness* **3** (3), 275 – 296

Greenhalgh T and Hurwitz B (1998) *Narrative-based Medicine: Dialogue and Discourse in Clinical Practice.* BMJ Books

Riessman C (1993) *Narrative Analysis.* London, Sage.

· 5 ·

RIGOUR IN QUALITATIVE RESEARCH

There appear to be two problems in assessing the rigour of qualitative research:

1. It has been judged by criteria which are well established in judging quantitative research, inappropriately in our view.
2. Qualitative methods have their origins in the social sciences, and criteria for judging work published in sociology journals have been used to judge work submitted to biomedical and primary care journals, again inappropriately in our view.

In 1995, the *British Medical Journal* published their checklist for establishing rigour in qualitative research. This focuses on:

- making the theoretical framework and methods explicit
- clear description of context
- justification of sampling strategy
- theoretical comprehensiveness of sampling strategy
- description of fieldwork and presentation of data
- description and theoretical justification of data analysis
- reliability of analysis
- use of quantitative evidence to test qualitative conclusions
- evidence of seeking potentially dissonant observations
- sufficient data to demonstrate relationship between interpretation and data.

For further reading see Article 14.

One way in which the reliability of analysis can be maximised is through **triangulation** – this should be integral to each stage of the research:

1. through the use of complementary sampling strategies, e.g. typical case and disconfirming case
2. through the use of complementary methods of data collection, e.g. observation and interviews

3. through the involvement of a multi-disciplinary panel in undertaking and reviewing data analysis, to ensure that no one set of interpretations is allowed to dominate.

However, a review of papers published in general practice suggests that there are more methodological questions than answers.

EXERCISE 11

Read Article 15.
What methodological questions are identified by Hoddinott and Pill?

Your answer should include the following points:
- *lack of contextual detail*
- *lack of methodological detail about the relationship between interviewer and interviewees*
- *the recruitment process*
- *explanation of research to respondents.*

Why are these methodological details important?

It is the explicit description of the research context, including the theoretical perspective of the researcher and methodological details, that allows qualitative studies to be assessed.

For a more detailed philosophical discussion of the concepts of validity and reliability, their roots in positivism, and their relevance for qualitative research, go back to Guba E and Lincoln (1994) and refer to Kirk J and Miller (1986).

In the social sciences, various alternative criteria for assessing qualitative research studies have been proposed. This includes the concepts of credibility and transferability in place of the notions of validity and generalisability, both familiar in quantitative research. For a review of this discussion see Murphy et al. (1998).

· 6 ·
CONCLUSION

WRITING UP QUALITATIVE RESEARCH

It is important to remember that in qualitative research it is the analytical framework developed from the data which provides the structure of a research report or journal paper. The paper should be an analytic account, not an account of respondents' narratives. The focus should be on describing the analytical process and results, rather than presenting a large quantity of pithy quotations. Data should be used to illustrate the analysis. The most reflective and insightful analyses use quotations sparingly whereas presenting a long list of data extracts tends to indicate that the data are under-analysed. Bear in mind the following:

Priorities

- describe the data collection process explicitly
- describe the process of analysis clearly
- concentrate on the results of the analysis
- present sufficient data to illustrate the analysis
- stay within the word count for the journal.

Pitfalls

- using qualitative terminology (e.g. **purposive**) without explanation
- too many data, and too little analysis
- referees who judge a qualitative paper from a quantitative perspective
- referees who judge a general practice paper from an exclusively sociological or biomedical perspective.

EXERCISE 12

Take a recent edition of one of your professional journals, and select a paper described as using qualitative methods.

How would you describe the presentation? Is the analytical method clear? Do data extracts support and illustrate the analysis?

FINALLY

Bear in mind the following before embarking on research:

Do

- be clear about your aims
- find an experienced qualitative researcher to advise/supervise your research
- find a peer group of researchers using similar methods
- read the literature in both primary care and social sciences journals
- plan data collection and analysis time (it can take several weeks to get transcripts from tapes)
- be practical: qualitative research is time consuming (one hour of interview time takes 5 – 6 hours to transcribe which costs approximately £50). Each hour of interview will take at least 10 hours of analysis time
- cost carefully.

Don't

- define your research area without reading relevant substantive and methodological literature (which may be in disciplines such as anthropology, sociology or psychology)
- start collecting data without reading the existing research
- start collecting data without thinking carefully about your own impact on the data
- collect data and then try to get help from a qualitative researcher
- underestimate the amount of time needed.

References
Baruch G (1981) Moral tales: parents' stories of encounters with the health professions. *Sociology of Health and Illness* **3** (3) 275 – 295

Bryman A and Burgess R (1994) *Analysing Qualitative Data.* London, Routledge

Denzin N and Lincoln Y (1994) *Handbook of Qualitative Research.* London, Sage

Dingwall R (1992) 'Don't mind him – he's from Barcelona': qualitative methods in health studies. In Daly J, Willis E and McDonald I (eds) *Researching Health Care.* London, Routledge

Glaser B (1978) *Theoretical sensitivity.* Mill Valley, CA: Sociology Press

Glaser B (1992) *Emergence vs. Forcing; Basics of Grounded Theory Analysis.* Mill Valley, CA, Sociology Press

Glaser B (1967) *The Discovery of Grounded Theory.* London, Weidenfeld & Nicholson

Granier S, Owen P, Pill R et al. (1998) Recognising meningococcal disease in primary care: qualitative study of how general practitioners process clinical and contextual information. *British Medical Journal* **316**, 276 – 9

Greenhalgh T and Hurwitz B (1998) *Narrative-based Medicine: Dialogue and Discourse in Clinical Practice.* BMJ Books

Greenhalgh T, Helman C and Chowdhury AM (1998a) Health beliefs and folk models of diabetes in British Bangladeshis: a qualitative study. *British Medical Journal* **316**, 978-83

Guba E and Lincoln Y (1994) Competing paradigms in qualitative research. In Denzin N and Lincoln Y (eds) *Handbook of Qualitative Research.* CA, Sage.

Janesick VJ (1994) The dance of qualitative research design: metaphor, methodolatry, and meaning in Denzin N and Lincoln Y (eds) *Handbook of Qualitative Research.* CA, Sage

Kai J (1996) What worries parents when their preschool children are acutely ill, and why: a qualitative study. *British Medical Journal* **313**, 983 – 6

Kirk J and Miller M (1986) *Reliability and Validity in Qualitative Research.* CA, Sage

Murphy E et al. (1998) Qualitative research methods in health technology assessment: a review of the literature HTA vol 2, no 16

Patton MQ (1990) *Qualitative Evaluation and Research Methods.* Newbury Park, CA, Sage

Riessman C (1993) *Narrative Analysis* p52. London, Sage

Ritchie J and Spencer L (1994) Qualitative data analysis for applied policy research. In Bryman A and Burgess R, *Analysing Qualitative Data.* London, Routledge

Silverman D (1993) *Interpreting Qualitative Data: Methods for Analysing Talk, Text and Interaction* p112. London, Sage

Strauss A (1987) *Qualitative Analysis for Social Scientists.* Cambridge, Cambridge University Press

Strauss A and Corbin J (1990) *Basics of Qualitative Research.* Newbury Park, CA, Sage

Tesch R (1990) *Qualitative Research: Analysis Types and Software Tools.* New York, Falmer Press

Suggested Further Reading
Baruch G (1981) Moral tales: parents' stories of encounters with the health professionals. *Sociology of Health and Illness* **3**(3), 275 – 295

Crabtree B and Miller W (1992) *Doing qualitative research* CA, Sage

Glaser B (1978) *Theoretical sensitivity.* Mill Valley, CA, Sociology Press

Glaser B (1992) *Emergence vs. Forcing; Basics of Grounded Theory Analysis.* Mill Valley, CA, Sociology Press

Glaser B (1967) *The Discovery of Grounded Theory.* London, Weidenfeld and Nicolson.

Janesick VJ (1994) The dance of qualitative research design: Metaphor, methodolatry, and meaning. In Denzin N and Lincoln Y (eds) *Handbook of Qualitative Research.* CA, Sage

Kirk J and Miller M (1986) *Reliability and Validity in Qualitative Research.* CA, Sage

Patton MQ (1990) *Qualitative Evaluation and Research Methods.* Newbury Park, CA, Sage

Riessman C (1993) *Narrative Analysis.* London, Sage

Ritchie J and Spencer L (1994) Qualitative data analysis for applied policy research. In Bryman A and Burgess R, *Analysing Qualitative Data.* London, Routledge

Strauss A (1987) *Qualitative Analysis for Social Scientists.* New York, Cambridge University Press

Strauss A and Corbin J (1990) *Basics of Qualitative Research.* London, Sage

Tesch R (1991) *Qualitative Research: Analysis Types and Software Tools.* London and Philadelphia, Falmer Press

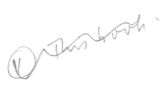

READING MATERIAL

1 WHAT IS QUALITATIVE RESEARCH?

1. Mathers N and Rowland (1997) General practice – a post-modern speciality? *British Journal of General Practice* **47**, 177 – 9.

2. Murphy E and Mattson B (1992) Qualitative research and family practice: a marriage made in heaven? *Family Practice* **9** (1), 85 – 91.

3. Guba E and Lincoln Y (1994) Competing paradigms in qualitative research. In Denzin N and Lincoln Y (eds) *Handbook of Qualitative Research*, CA, Sage.

4. Granier S, Owen P, Pill R et al. (1998) Recognising meningococcal disease in primary care: qualitative study of how general practitioners process clinical and contextual information. *British Medical Journal* **316**, 276 – 9.

5. Greenhalgh T, Helman C and Chowdhury AM (1998) Health beliefs and folk models of diabetes in British Bangladeshis: a qualitative study. *British Medical Journal* **316**, 978 – 83.

6. Kai J (1996) What worries parents when their preschool children are acutely ill, and why: a qualitative study. *British Medical Journal* **313**, 983 – 6.

2 METHODS OF DATA COLLECTION

7. Britten N (1995) Qualitative interviews in medical research. *British Medical Journal* **311**, 251 – 3.

8. Kitzinger J (1995) Introducing focus groups. *British Medical Journal* **311**, 299 – 302.

9. Mays C and Pope N (1995) Observational methods in health care settings. *British Medical Journal* **311**, 182 – 4.

10. Fitzpatrick R and Boulton M (1994) Qualitative methods for assessing health care. *Quality in Health Care* **3**, 107 – 113.

11. Silverman D (1993) *Interpreting Qualitative Data: Methods for Analysing Talk, Text and Interaction*, London, Sage.

3 SAMPLING

12. Patton MQ (1990) Designing qualitative studies in *Qualitative Evaluation and Research Methods*, CA, Sage.

4 DATA ANALYSIS

13. Bryman A and Burgess R (1994) *Analysing Qualitative Data*. London, Routledge.

5 ACCURACY IN QUALITATIVE RESEARCH

14. Mays C and Pope N (1995) Rigour and qualitative research. *British Medical Journal* **311**, 109 – 112.

15. Hoddinott P and Pill R (1997) A review of recently published qualitative research in general practice. More methodological questions than answers? *Family Practice* **14** (4), 313 – 19.

SECTION 1

SECTION 2

SECTION 3

SECTION 4

SECTION 5

ARTICLE 1

This Article was first published in the British Journal of General Practice and is reproduced by permission of the British Journal of General Practice

GENERAL PRACTICE – A POST-MODERN SPECIALTY?

Nigel Mathers • Stephen Rowland

N Mathers, BSC, MBCHB, MD, PHD, MRCGP, Senior lecturer, Institute of General Practice, University of Sheffield;

S Rowland, MA, MED, FRSA, Senior lecturer in education, University of Sheffield.

Submitted: 25 March 1996; accepted: 1 November 1996.

British Journal of General Practice 1997 **47**, 177-179

SUMMARY

The 'modern' view of the world is based on the premise that we can discover the essential truth of the world using scientific method. The assumption is made that knowledge so acquired has been 'uncontaminated' by the mind of the investigator. Post-modern theory, however, is concerned with the process of knowing and how our minds are part of the process, i.e. our perceptions of reality and the relationships between different concepts are important influences on our ways of knowing. The values of post-modern theory are those of uncertainty, many different voices and experiences of reality and multifaceted descriptions of truth. These values are closer to our experience of general practice than the 'modern' values of scientific rationalism and should be reflected in a new curriculum for general practice.

Keywords: theoretical models; curriculum; randomized controlled trials.

INTRODUCTION

'How are things at home?' the student asked the patient. 'Fine' the patient replied. The student struggled. 'Um . . . tell me who lives with you?' he asked. When presenting this incident later, the student recited a list of people with all their ages and occupations. He was rather pleased with himself and his ability to take a 'full social and psychological history'. However, he was unable to show any sensitive understanding of the patient in her context or what the illness might mean to this patient. This is the problem. Sometimes, when we try and teach our students or registrars how to take a social and psychological history in general practice, they may persist in using such an inappropriate biomedical or teaching hospital model to elicit the information. Indeed, the problem is even wider in that trying to design an appropriate curriculum for general practice is extremely difficult. Not only are we sometimes unsure what 'good' general practice is,[1] but also what is an appropriate model for general practice to teach and how it might be best learnt by our students.

The current curriculum for general practice has, to a large extent, gradually evolved over the years by 'plugging the gaps' in the main medical school teaching. For example, academic departments of general practice are usually responsible for the teaching of communication skills. The difficulty has been not only in defining what exactly we mean by the discipline of general practice but also how we can establish our credentials as a 'serious' academic subject alongside the major medical specialties of medicine and surgery. As one dean suggested to one of the authors (NM) recently: 'You have managed to create a "dog's breakfast" out of service provision.' The infamous comment of the 1960s that general practice is the repository of those who 'have fallen off the ladder' with no particular claims to either special knowledge or an academic specialty in its own right is alive and well in medical schools up and down the country! Clearly, with the growing importance of primary care in the National Health Service and increasing amounts of undergraduate teaching in the community, we need to think carefully about what a curriculum for general practice should contain and how it should be delivered.

A 'modern' approach to curriculum design would suggest that all that needs to be done to prepare a curriculum for general practice is to define the:

- aims and objectives
- content
- process
- assessment and evaluation.

And the rest is a question of resources! Much effort has been devoted to this, but there remains the problem of what we mean by general practice. A further difficulty is that this approach is based on a 'scientific' model of general practice, and this way of thinking can lead to the problem described at the beginning of this article. A curriculum designed in this rather mechanistic (or biomedical) way is very limited in that, for example, it does not allow for the dynamic and continuous influence of evaluation on planning, or indeed for any differences between the 'planned' curriculum, the 'taught' curriculum and the 'learnt' curriculum.[2] The process of curriculum design may alternatively be regarded as essentially a form of applied philosophy[3] with the major concern being conceptual analysis. The prime purpose of studying the curriculum is to 'achieve conceptual clarity in thinking about the curriculum as a basis for ensuring practical coherence in the implementation of that thinking'.

A quest for a satisfactory curriculum for general practice leads on from here to the necessity for an appropriate matching of both theory and practice.

A NEW CURRICULUM FOR GENERAL PRACTICE?

The 'modern' view of the world is based on the premise that we can discover the essential truth of 'out there' (i.e. outside of our minds) using scientific method. Our certainty that we have discovered the 'real truth' about the world is based on the rigour of the scientific method that has been used. A randomized clinical trial (RCT), for example, gives us the best approximation of what is 'really happening' and can support a cause and effect relationship between an intervention and an outcome. The assumption is made, however, that the knowledge so acquired has been unmediated or 'uncontaminated' by the mind of the investigator. This is the evidence-based approach to general practice, and those of us who work in the 'swampy lowlands' of everyday practice rather than the 'sunny uplands' of academia recognize that this is fine as far as it goes, however, this is not very far, and such an approach has very limited application in our day-to-day work, concerned as it is with managing illness in context. This can create very real difficulties for both doctors and students as they struggle to apply such a model that does not very often or necessarily fit. A different and complementary way of looking at our work is necessary if we are to achieve an appropriate matching of theory and practice for a curriculum that truly reflects the 'real' world of general practice and introduces our students to it.

POST-MODERNISM AND THE CURRICULUM

Post-modern theory is difficult to explain. The word post-modern itself comes from the Latin meaning 'after just now', so in one sense everything that is happening now is post modern. However, the theory itself is a consequence of the twentieth century's obsession with language and is rooted in structuralism, which is a school of formal linguistics. In a nutshell, the theory originated with the premise that you cannot stand outside language to understand it. Post-modernism is concerned with the process of knowing and how our minds are part of that process. Our perceptions of reality and the relationships between different concepts are important influences on our ways of knowing. Derrida[4] wrote about presence, meaning that the status of any knowledge that we claim as true is true because of the process we have used to come to know it. In other words, the knowledge we gain using an RCT, for example, has presence because we believe that such a method gives us access to the underlying truth of the world, i.e. an objective reality. It is this belief that is

important, described in post-modern theory as the scientific discourse. However, beliefs do not arise in isolation, and scientific discourse is rooted within the social community of scientists. Post-modern theory states that such a discourse (and there are others) is based on power (the ability to claim presence) and knowledge (the presence that is claimed).

The other component of post-modern theory that is necessary to understand is the idea of difference. Since we are always constrained by our perceptions, any description of underlying reality is a reflection of its difference from other things rather than its essence.[5] Language can only convey meaning in this way. We know what something is because of what it is not. Diabetes, for example, can only be recognized and known as diabetes because we can contrast it with a central concept of health (i.e. not diabetes). This idea of difference means that the harder we try to define precisely what we mean by a concept, the more it slips away from our definition. Indeed, any definition we try to make of the 'underlying truth' of a concept can only be understood in relation to everything else. A description of reality, therefore, is only ever a changing approximation, and however hard we try to make it 'more real' by particular methodologies, the more it slips from our grasp.[6]

What might this mean for a general practice curriculum? Hopefully, it is clear from the above that the values of post-modern theory are those of uncertainty, many different voices and experiences of reality, and multifaceted descriptions of 'truth'. This, it seems to us, is closer to the values and experience of general practice than the 'modern' values of a 'scientific' rationalism. It also clarifies why such a biomedical model does not seem to 'fit' our daily reality and why our students have such difficulty in crossing the 'cultural divide' from secondary to primary care. A post-modern approach to a curriculum for general practice would therefore consider the claims of our current curriculum to presence and reflect on the themes of power (what the basis is for the ability to claim presence) and knowledge (what counts as a valid model).

TOWARDS A POST-MODERN CURRICULUM FOR GENERAL PRACTICE

This article has given a brief overview of some of the post-modern ideas that might underlie a new curriculum for general practice. To define such a curriculum is, in post-modern terms, almost a contradiction. However, we can consider how a curriculum could be related to our current teaching and practice, and how this knowledge is affected by general practice's claims to both power and knowledge.

One of the authors (NM) recently attended the Annual Scientific Meeting of the Association of University Departments of General Practice (AUDGP) in Newcastle. A great deal of high-quality scientific work was presented. However, 'high quality' tended to be synonymous with a 'modern' model of scientific endeavour. For example, an RCT comparison of out-of-hours care provided by the deputizing service and own-practice doctors was presented, and a fine, elegant study this was. However, the danger is that RCTs can sometimes be used to answer only relatively trivial questions in primary care. Indeed, in some cases the questions asked in general practice using such a model have been severely constrained or even 'driven' by the methodology. The chosen design may result in the 'wrong' questions being asked. Such a claim to 'presence' based on a 'modern' claim to knowledge, and a claim to power based on the emulation of secondary care methodology can only play one part in a post-modern curriculum for general practice.

Other sessions at the AUDGP presented results from more qualitative studies. Here, general practice's claim to presence was associated with a more subjective model – 'soft' rather than 'hard' science. The rigour of the methodology enabled a claim to knowledge to be made. Such claims, however, can sit uneasily with doctors whose training has been based on the traditional biomedical model. GPs have a natural distrust of claims based on such 'soft' methods and can find difficulty in incorporating such knowledge in practice.

Some studies presented were particularly concerned with evaluating educational initiatives, and the difficulties of producing 'high-quality' educational research were discussed. These educational initiatives assumed a training model as a basis for claims to knowledge and power, and the focus was more on process than content – such an approach to the teaching of general practice may be rather more appropriate to a post-modern curriculum.

Schön[7] has attempted to define a reflective or critical model for the teaching of professional practice. He cites the widespread disillusion with the professional 'experts' and their objectivist philosophy that focuses on the technical and the testable, and separates the ends from the means, yet fails to train for the real problems of practice. He suggests a model for professional practice based on reflection both in and on practice. Such claims to power and knowledge would be appropriate for a post-modern curriculum in which the knowing is in the doing. The process consists of problem setting and problem solving.

Problem setting in general practice is the process by which we name the problem we wish to consider or the question we wish to ask and define the context in which it should be answered. This involves, for example, the use of 'critical incidents' in the curriculum. Problem solving is a reflective conversation whereby a unique and uncertain situation comes to be understood through the attempt to change it, and changed through the attempt to understand it in conjunction with peers and general practice tutors.

The educational values of a curriculum based on such a reflective or critical model of professional practice would be practical, active and pragmatic, and could encompass all the current models of general practice. The implied teaching methods of this model, such as practical attachments ('apprenticeship') and small group teaching, would be more appropriate than didactic lectures. Methods of assessment would be mainly by portfolios, projects, continual assessment, competencies and peer review rather than MCQs and OSCEs. The factual overload identified by the GMC[8] in *Tomorrow's Doctors* would be reduced. In addition, the curriculum would have 'street credibility' with the majority of GPs, since it would be based in the 'real world' – the 'swampy lowlands' of everyday practice where chaos and uncertainty are ever present!

Many observers believe that a 'paradigm shift' is now overdue in medical practice and education. James Willis[9] is one such author. In his book, *The Paradox of Progress*[9], he writes: 'We understand the world we live in more completely than we have ever done before, and yet we understand it less'.

References

1. Toon P. What is good general practice? [Occasional Paper No. 65.] London: Royal College of General Practitioners, 1994.
2. Lowry S. Medical education. London: BMJ Publishing Group, 1993.
3. Kelly AV. The curriculum: theory and practice. (3rd edn.) London: Chapman & Hall, 1989.
4. Derrida J. Of grammatology. Baltimore, MD, USA: Johns Hopkins University Press, 1976.
5. Lemert C. General social theory, irony, postmodernism. In: Postmodernism and social theory. Seidman S, Wagner D (eds). Oxford: Blackwell, 1992.
6. Fox N. Postmodernism, sociology and health. Buckingham: Open University Press, 1993.
7. Schön DA. The crisis of professional knowledge, and the pursuit of an epistemology of practice. J Interprof Care 1992; **6**: 49-63.
8. General Medical Council (GMC). Tomorrow's doctors. London: GMC, 1993.
9. Willis J. The paradox of progress. Oxford: Radcliffe Medical Press, 1995.

Address for correspondence
Dr Nigel Mathers, Department of General Practice, Community Sciences Centre, Northern General Hospital, Herries Road, Sheffield S5 7AU.

This Article was first published in Family Practice (Oxford University Press) and is reproduced by permission of Oxford University Press

QUALITATIVE RESEARCH AND FAMILY PRACTICE: A MARRIAGE MADE IN HEAVEN?

Elizabeth Murphy and Bengt Mattson

Elizabeth Murphy • School of Social Studies, University of Nottingham, UK and
Bengt Mattson • University of Umeå, Sweden.
Correspondence to: Elizabeth Murphy, School of Social Studies, University of Nottingham, University Park, Nottingham NG7 2RD, UK.

Family Practice 1992 9: 85–91.

ARTICLE 2

Recent years have seen the development of interest in the usefulness of qualitative methods in family practice research. This paper shows how the underlying concerns of family practice medicine parallel those of the qualitative research tradition. After contrasting the philosophical underpinnings of both quantitative and qualitative methods, we go on to describe the methodological commitments of qualitative research. We relate this emerging debate within family practice to that which has taken place in other disciplines, particularly that of education. We discuss the relative strengths of qualitative and quantitative methods, and argue that these two traditions have complementary contributions to make to the discipline of family practice medicine.

INTRODUCTION

The emergence of family practice as an academic discipline has been associated with a growing awareness of its distinctive features, when compared with other medical specialities. The distribution of problems presented to family practitioners differs from that experienced by their hospital colleagues. It is estimated[1] that of those who consult in general practice, 50% have no identifiable pathology, 35% have self-limiting disease conditions and 15% have disease which requires active treatment. Many of the health problems presented in family practice are those which Balint termed 'undifferentiated'.[2] Family practitioners take responsibility for the total health care of individuals and families, and therefore their primary focus is upon the individual rather than the disease entity.[3] In family practice the patient is treated, at least in principle, as a subject rather than an object.[4,5] The presenting complaints and the patients themselves can be considered in the context of their family and community lives.[3,6,7] Family practitioners will often be more concerned with care than with cure.[1] In McWhinney's view, family practitioners attach importance to the subjective aspects of medicine, both in terms of understanding the patient's perspective and an awareness that their own feelings and values will influence the way in which they practice medicine.[3]

Appropriate Methodologies for Family Practice Research

Given the distinctive concerns of family practice medicine, the appropriateness of operating exclusively within a research tradition derived from the hospital specialities has been questioned.[8-10] This questioning has been linked to a growing awareness of the particular relevance of social science research to family practice medicine,[11] and the resultant encounters with a broader range of methodologies. We argue, in this paper, that qualitative methodologies may have a particular relevance to family practice research, because they share many of the commitments of family medicine as outlined above.

Qualitative methodologies continue to be under-represented in family practice research. There has, however, been some evidence of an upsurge in interest in such methods. A review of the articles published in *Family Practice* during 1989 and 1990 reveals that 16% have at least some element which could be described as qualitative. With a few notable exceptions[12-14] the tendency has been for researchers in family medicine, to 'add on' a qualitative element to what is primarily a quantitative study. The continued reluctance to carry out thorough going qualitative research can partly be explained by the time-consuming nature of such research, and the lack of expertise in using such methods.[10] It may also reflect an anxiety about whether traditional sources of funding for medical research would welcome proposals using qualitative methodologies. However, we believe that reluctance to make use of qualitative methods in family practice research is also the result of a failure to understand the theoretical and philosophical background to these methodologies. It may also partly reflect a desire to be seen to be doing research which is methodologically orthodox as perceived by academics in other medical disciplines. Balint[2] would no doubt have characterized this as part of the 'perpetuation of the teacher-pupil relationship' between hospital consultants and family practice doctors.

The range of research questions which needs to be addressed in relation to family practice is very wide. We would argue that some of these clearly warrant investigation using traditional quantitative methodologies derived from the natural sciences. For example, if one is investigating the impact upon referral rates of making a particular diagnostic test available to family practitioners, with a view to assessing the resource implications, it would seem appropriate to design an experimental intervention using quantitative techniques. If on the other hand, one is interested in understanding the process of referral, either as an end in itself, or as a basis for developing educational initiatives to modify referral behaviour, qualitative methodologies may be more useful.

We believe, therefore, that, to exploit its full potential, family practice research needs to make use of the widest possible range of research methodologies. The principle to be applied in choosing a particular method should be that of 'fitness for the purpose' rather than traditional orthodoxy. Cronbach makes the same point in relation to investigations in another research area, that of education, where he advocates 'maximally useful designs'.[15] 'Most writings on design suggest that an investigation is to be judged by its form, and certain forms are held up as universal ideals. In contrast, I would argue that investigations have functions and that a form highly suitable for one investigation would not be appropriate for the next'.

We believe that both quantitative and qualitative methods have strengths as well as weaknesses, and the choice of method always involves a 'trade off' between these.

Quantitative research has traditionally reflected a positivistic, philosophical orientation, while qualitative researchers have generally looked to an alternative tradition. We argue that this alternative tradition, described below, is congruent with many of the commitments of family practice medicine, and that, for this reason alone, researchers in this discipline could usefully explore the appropriateness of the methods associated with it.

In contrasting the theoretical preoccupations of positivism and anti-positivism there is danger of creating an artificial philosophical gulf between quantitative and qualitative methods, by suggesting that they are the expression of competing and essentially irreconcilable methodological paradigms. In reality, for us, the choice of qualitative or quantitative methods is a technical matter, which should be dictated by the nature of the research question, rather than the result of epistemological debate.[16] However, we believe that an understanding of the philosophical tradition and methodological concerns towards which qualitative research has traditionally looked, will offer a more appropriate basis for the evaluation of such work than that which has generally been applied to it within the discipline of family practice.

In attempting to describe the theoretical basis of both quantitative and qualitative methods, we are also conscious of the risk of gross generalization and over-simplification. We recognize that in characterizing what we see to be the central commitments of each approach we will fail to do justice to the complexity of the subject and are forced to ignore those, for example, who have combined positivism and qualitative methods or anti-positivism and quantitative methods.

Positivism and its Implications for Research Methods

Positivism is a somewhat ambiguous term, but there are some basic characteristics of this tradition which can be identified.[16,17] One of the central commitments of positivism is that conventional natural science research methods should be the model for all social research. By this it is implied that the logic of the experiment is the only acceptable logic for scientific research and that only knowledge acquired in this way is 'scientific' knowledge.

A second commitment of positivism relates to the type of explanation which is deemed appropriate for science. All explanation should take the form of 'covering laws'.[16,17] This is to say that the researcher is aiming to establish general laws of the kind which are found in physics. The value of such laws is that they not only allow us to explain phenomena in retrospect, but they also permit us to predict what will happen in the future. In fact it is difficult to think of any laws which allow us to predict clinical outcome with the precision of physical laws. However, this is the 'gold standard' towards which medical researchers conventionally strive.

Lastly, positivism is committed to the view that only observable phenomena can be accepted as knowledge. Hence unless feelings, motivations, attitudes and so on can be rendered observable in some way, they cannot be accepted as knowledge.

Against the background of these philosophical commitments, the hypothetico-deductive method has been enshrined as the cornerstone of medical research, and hypothesis testing as the legitimate preoccupation of scientific studies. Clearly the testing of hypotheses is an important goal for family practice research. However, we believe that the model is an inappropriately constraining strait-jacket into which to force many of the issues which general practice wishes to address. To limit the research topics which can be legitimately posed in family practice to those which are open to the hypothetico-deductive method is to deny the discipline access to other significant sources of knowledge.

The rise of positivism and the logic of the experiment have been crucial developments in the emergence of scientific clinical practice based upon rational and scientific principles. Cochrane[18] rightly emphasizes the central importance of the randomized controlled clinical trial for the assessment of therapeutic interventions. The emphasis upon clinical objectivity, quantitative measurements and the control of extraneous variables are all important in assessing the usefulness of particular treatments. Such research methodology is rightly preoccupied with the issues of representativeness, validity and reliability of measurements. Nevertheless, as Dudley[19] has pointed out, there are dangers inherent in the unthinking elevation of the randomized controlled trial to a position where it is the only acceptable means of obtaining reliable knowledge.

Alternatives to Positivism

In recent years tentative interest in the applicability to family practice research of non-positivistic approach has begun to be voiced in Britain,[9,20] Australia[8], Scandanavia[21] and the USA.[10] The contribution which non-positivistic approaches have to offer to general practice is under discussion, and this has been associated with an upsurge of interest in qualitative methodologies. In some quarters they have been greeted with scepticism while in others they have been seen as an attractive alternative to the constraints of quantitative approaches. The previous emphasis upon standardization of measurement has come to be seen by some as limiting the possibility of researching the diverse and contradictory realities of patients and their doctors. Blind application of reductionist methods may lead to the execution of elegant experiments contributing little to questions of importance because the soluble is not necessarily the important, or because the imposition of experimental conditions can lead to findings which are irrelevant to practice.

Family practice researchers are not alone in this sense of frustration. In education, nursing research and the social sciences it has resulted in the development of a distinct, yet complementary qualitative research tradition which has been thriving for several decades[16,22-26] The messianic enthusiasm for quantitative methods which followed the development of modern statistical techniques in the middle years of this century,[6] has given way to an awareness of the need to combine both qualitative and quantitative methodologies. Professor John Nisbet, a leading commentator on the debates that occurred in educational research in the 1970s, provides a useful retrospective view of this development in education. In his address to the inaugural meeting of the British Educational Research Association, in 1974, he reflected upon the relationship between the newly emerging qualitative research methods and traditional approaches:[27] 'We are often presented with this style of research as a challenge to the traditional model. To some extent it is; but my position is that no one of these styles is 'right', and none is altogether 'wrong'. The most effective research employs a variety of strategies, across the spectrum'.

However, if we are to integrate qualitative methods into our research practice, it must be in the context of understanding them in their own terms. We must not simply criticize them because they do not fit into established positivistic structures. These methods are related to a different philosophical tradition and are best equipped to address different research questions, and often provide fundamentally different types of answer.

This tradition challenges the appropriateness of natural science as a model for all research. In particular it is argued that where research is concerned with understanding people as social beings, as opposed to people as machines, natural science is an inappropriate reference point. Whereas positivists view behaviour as the outcome of internal or external forces, which are to be investigated by the researcher as a detached, neutral observer, the qualitative tradition emphasizes that people actively interpret the world in which they live and the experiences which they have. Behaviour is seen not simply as the outcome of determining variables, but as arising from the individual's interpretation of events and experiences.[28]

The crucial factor in explaining an individual's conscious acts is seen to be the meaning which (s)he attributes to events or experiences. Natural science can demonstrate that metal responds to heat by expanding, whatever the cause of that heat is. Likewise, at least in general, people respond to excessive heat by sweating, irrespective of their interpretation of that heat. However, conscious acts associated with extreme heat, such as the removal of clothing, are not governed solely by physiological changes in response to heat. They may also be governed by considerations of modesty, expectations about future activity, such as going outside, pride in a new sweater, and so on. It is argued therefore that when we are seeking to understand people as social beings, rather than as a series of physiological responses, something different from the positivistic approach is helpful.

Advocates of this tradition, therefore, argue that covering-law models are inappropriate for understanding the social world. Rather they call for 'explanation by understanding',[16] where what is of interest are the motives, reasons and so on which lie behind actions. The emphasis is not so much upon prediction, as on being able to make actions intelligible, given the way in which the individual or group makes sense of the situation. There is an emphasis therefore on understanding the culture of the particular people one is studying – in the tradition of anthropology.[23]

Researchers drawing upon this tradition argue that we cannot hope to understand the social world by simply studying artificial simulations of it in experiments or structured interviews. A central preoccupation of social research must be to study how particular groups behave in real life situations.

Methodological Implications of Anti-positivism

The term 'qualitative research' includes a range of different methodological approaches and it is beyond the scope of this paper to describe the nuances of each approach. For the sake of clarity, in discussing the methodological commitments arising from this alternative tradition, we have therefore chosen to present those which characterize one particular branch of qualitative research, that of ethnography.[23]

Within ethnography, there is an emphasis upon description. Whereas quantitative researchers emphasize the importance of testing hypotheses, ethnographers have traditionally stressed the value of rigorous description. It is not so much that ethnographers deny the importance of explanation – of answering the 'why?' question. It is rather that they consider it premature to ask 'why?' when one doesn't yet have the answer to the 'what?' question. This emphasis on rigorous description was of course one of the hallmarks of the early anatomists and pathologists who were the early medical scientists.[29] It could be argued that just as adequate description was an essential forerunner of hypothesis testing research in these fields, so too it needs to be established as the bedrock of future study of the social dimensions of clinical practice.

The emphasis therefore is on discovery. This in part arises from ethnography's roots in cultural anthropology, where researchers set out to understand primitive cultures. The dangers of 'ethnocentrism' or judging all human action from the standpoint of one's own culture, were very obvious to such anthropologists and the 'good anthropologist' was seen as attempting to put their preconceptions to one side, and studying the chosen society in its own terms. This emphasis has been carried over into studies in our own culture and ethnographers attempt to 'enter the culture' of those they study. In practical terms this means that the researchers try not to impose their thinking, about how things are, upon the researched. Unlike the quantitative researchers who may have developed a standardized questionnaire before approaching their subjects, operationalizing predetermined variables in a way which reflects their own understanding of what is important, what is significant and how things ought to be, ethnographers will try to assume a naive stance in relation to the people they are studying. Ethnographers aim to provide a context in which people can display their own thinking rather than asking them to constrain their thinking to fit a preconceived schema. The ethnographer will avoid imposing prior and potentially inappropriate frames of reference on those they study. Douglas[3] uses satire to contrast this qualitative approach with more traditional interview methods: "How much more proud and worthy—serenely confident and powerful—we feel when we can impose the structure of discourse and of reality itself upon our little 'subjects': 'Sit there 'subject'. Now, here is a questionnaire with five hundred questions on it. They are written in stone and encompass the entire realm of possible questions concerning these realities. There are only five possible responses to each one. All you have to do is meekly indicate for each of my preconceived computer-card holes where your peg fits—that and absolutely nothing more. Then be gone with you."

In practical terms ethnography's commitment to discovery leads to an emphasis upon a research strategy which is relatively open and unstructured. The researcher is unlikely to decide in advance what precisely is to be studied, within a particular context. He or she is much more open than the quantitative researcher to following up unexpected leads which arise from the research.

For example, in carrying out research to inform the planning of educational packages about diet, for use with people who have diabetes, the quantitative researcher might develop a test of knowledge about the diabetic diet, where the questions would reflect the concerns of current medical models of dietary management in diabetes. From this information the researcher could identify the 'gaps' in lay knowledge and plan educational interventions accordingly. The ethnographer is more likely to set out to discover the complexity of lay beliefs

about diet, the significance which particular types of food, or patterns of eating, have for individuals. This information might be sought in the context of less researcher-dominated interactions with patients, where the ethnographer would encourage the patient to talk freely about food, without imposing the constraints of a pre-structured questionnaire. Such discoveries might enable planners to identify dietary recommendations which are compatible with both lay and medical models of 'good diet'. Alternatively knowledge of the significance which certain types of food have for individuals would permit the design of educational materials which address the conflicts between lay and medical thinking.

There is is also an emphasis within ethnography on generating theory.[31] In quantitative research there is considerable stress upon testing theory, but perhaps less attention to where such theory comes from. Sometimes the hypothesis is the product of a painstaking research process where each step points inexorably to the next hypothesis to be tested. Sometimes, it is based on 'armchair theorizing', where the researcher draws upon his experience to speculate about what the world might be like and constructs a hypothesis based upon that. The alternative, proposed by stenographers, is that hypotheses should arise from data, and should follow from the rigorous description discussed above.

Again, in ethnography, there is an emphasis upon uncovering the meanings and interpretations which lie behind behaviour. There is a commitment to seeing the world through the eyes of the people who are being studied. In practical terms this demands a willingness to empathize with those being studied, and a commitment to penetrating the frames of meaning with which they operate. This is a direct result of the rejection of the 'covering-law' approach advocated by positivists. The etlinographer is concerned to understand behaviour in the terms of those who are behaving, rather than seeing it as the outcome of specific variables such as gender, social class and personality traits.

Ethnographers also emphasize the importance of understanding behaviour in context, or holistically, believing that the actions of individuals must be seen in relation to what is going on at a more general level, and cannot wholly be understood apart from that.

Traditionally ethnographers have been greatly concerned about naturalism. They have argued that social life must be studied, as far as possible, as it occurs. They criticize quantitative researchers for creating artificial situations and argue that this artificiality distorts the findings of such research. Ethnographers therefore try to minimize their own impact upon the setting and to find as far as possible a natural role for themselves. Obviously, at one level this is naive, in that we always affect situations of which we are part.[23,24] A more sophisticated approach to this problem is that of reflexivity so that the researcher consciously monitors and reflects upon the impact which (s)he has upon a setting.

In general ethnography emphasizes description of the qualities of a phenomenon, rather than the counting of the amount of a quality that exists, or the number of people who have a particular quality. An example from research recently published in the *British Medical Journal* will illustrate this point. Coulter *et al.*[32] analysed 18754 referrals from 127 GPs to hospital specialists. Each doctor was asked to choose between 7 preformulated reasons for referral. These were:

for a specified investigation (diagnosis reasonably clear); for treatment or operation (diagnosis known); for advice on management and referral back (diagnosis known); for specialist to take over management (diagnosis known); for a second opinion to reassure them (GP) that they had done all that was required; for a second opinion to reassure patients or their families that they (the GP) had done all that was required; for other reasons.

This piece of research is firmly grounded in the quantitative tradition. The concern is to apply preformulated categories and to count. An ethnographer approaching the same area would avoid the imposition of such categories in advance and might attempt to discover from the individual GPs what they believed motivated them to make particular referrals. The reality would undoubtedly be much more complex than this study implies. It would allow room for the observation that 'I referred this patient because the last one I had with these symptoms died unexpectedly', or 'I referred this patient because I was tired and didn't want to argue.'

This example demonstrates the relative strengths of qualitative and quantitative approaches. Lee Cronbach, a well-known quantitative methodologist, described the complementarity of the two approaches. Quantitative methodologies allow the researcher to put forward generalizations, while qualitative methodologies may allow us to supply the detail which explains the cases in which these generalizations do not hold.[33] 'Instead of making generalizations the ruling consideration in our research, I suggest that we reverse our priorities. An observer collecting data in one particular situation is in a position to appraise a practice or proposition in that setting, observing effects in context'.

Much of conventional thinking about research design came from agricultural research studies where various experimental interventions were evaluated in relation to such outcome measures as crop yield. Stenhouse contrasted the concerns of education with those of agricultural science to demonstrate how a methodology based upon probability which was adequate within agriculture was less so when applied to education. He argued that education is concerned with individuals, and the fate of individuals, rather than that of populations.[34] 'While in agriculture it is normally accepted that the fate of individual seeds of corn or individual battery hens does not matter unless it makes the relation of investment to gross yield unfavourable, in education the fate of individual students is generally held to be an appropriate concern. Furthermore, while in agriculture it was generally assumed that the expense of differentiating treatments between individuals could

only be justified in clinical cases on expensive animals, in education it is widely believed that the treatment of students should be a differential response to diagnostic assessments of their needs'. This concern to tailor management to the needs of the individual is surely a key feature of family practice medicine, and research which will help to inform the management of cases which do not fit generalizations is surely an appropriate activity within that discipline.

A further emphasis within ethnography has been summed up as 'multiple perspectives'. This again goes back to the roots of ethnography in cultural anthropology. Anthropologists insisted that the so-called primitive people they studied should not be treated as superstitious or mentally inferior to Westerners but should be understood as adopting equally rational, though not necessarily factually correct, world views. Likewise ethnographers in our own society start from a position of respecting those they research, and assuming that whatever they do is a rational response to their situation, in the light of the information available to them and the assumptions with which they operate.

Congruence of Qualitative Methods and Family Practice

The principles of qualitative research do, we believe, reflect many of the concerns of family medicine. Both are concerned with treating people as social beings rather than as the 'carriers of disease'. Both are concerned with the meaning of certain events or symptoms to those individuals who experience them. Both stress the importance of understanding the individual within his own context and both are concerned with individuals as 'wholes' rather than reducing them to the sum of their parts. We argue therefore, that qualitative research methods are particularly appropriate for use in family practice research, and that to neglect their potential is to do a disservice to our discipline.

The use of qualitative methods in family practice research has pragmatic as well as philosophical appeal. The choice of methodology is always a trade off between the strengths and weaknesses of available approaches. Qualitative methods pose particular problems in terms both of the the interpretation of data and generalisation from it. The very richness and diversity of qualitative data, which is one of its strengths, often inhibits the tight specification of variables and the possibility of establishing relationships between them. On the other hand, qualitative methods are ideally suited to the development of explanations and hypotheses. They minimize artificiality and offer the researcher maximum flexibility in reformulating the question in the course of research, or adapting sampling procedures to enhance the developing analysis. Such methods give access to data which may be extremely difficult for researchers in other traditions to access. They are often more effective in sensitive situations, and are more likely to give access to an understanding of people's 'private' as opposed to 'public' worlds.[35]

ARTICLE 2

Concluding Remarks

As discussed above, in other disciplines, such as education, the debate about the relative merits of qualitative and quantitative methods has persisted for more than two decades. In the initial stages this debate was marked by considerable polarization and acrimony. In recent years there has been some degree of rapprochement and an emphasis upon the integration of the two traditions. It would be unfortunate if the development of qualitative methods in family practice were to be characterized by the degree of hostility observed elsewhere. We believe that qualitative and quantitative methods are complementary approaches to the research issues generated in family practice, and that, both individually and in combination, they have much to contribute to our discipline. Any such co-operation and collaboration must be built upon an adequate understanding of both traditions, and we offer this introduction to the methodological commitments of family research as a contribution to that development.

To leave the security of orthodox methods and to take the risk of adopting innovative approaches is no easy undertaking. Nevertheless, if, as we have argued, qualitative methods have a distinctive and important contribution to make to the knowledge base of family practice, then we ignore them at our peril. As Soren Kierkegaard has said, 'To dare is to lose foothold for a little while-not to dare is to lose oneself.'[36]

Acknowledgements

The authors wish to acknowledge the support and stimulation of colleagues at the Department of Primary Medical Care, at the University of Southampton, and in particular the thoughtful comments which Dr Ann Louise Kinmonth made on an earlier draft of this paper. We are also grateful to Professor Roger Murphy for helpful discussions about the parallels between research in education and family practice, and to the Department of General Practice, at the University of Nottingham, where Elizabeth Murphy was a visiting Research Fellow during the writing of this paper.

Elizabeth Murphy was supported during the writing of this paper by the Economic and Social Research Council.

References

[1] Kusher T. Doctor-patient relationships in general practice—a different model. J *Med Ethics* 1981; 7: 128–131.

[2] Balint M. *The doctor, his patient and the illness.* London: Pitman, 1957.

[3] McWhinney IR. *A textbook of family medicine.* Oxford: Oxford University Press, 1989.

[4] Marinker M. The chameleon, the Judas goat and the cuckoo. *J R Coll Gen Pract* 1978; **28**:199–206.

[5] Rainsberry RPN. Values, paradigms and research in family medicine. *Earn Pract* 1986; **3**: 209–215.

[6] Gordon MJ. Research traditions available to family medicine. *JFam Pract* 1978; 7: 59–68.

[7] Helman CG. The role of context in primary care. *J R Coll Gen Pract* 1984; **34**: 546–550.

[8] Underwood P, Gray D, Winkler R., Cutting open Newton's apple to find the cause of gravity: a reply to Julian Tudor Hart. *Br Med J* 1985; **291**: 1322–1325.

[9] Aldridge D, Pietroni P. Research trials in general practice: towards a focus on clinical practice. *Fam Pract* 1987; **4**: 311–315.

[10] Kuzel AJ. Naturalistic inquiry: An appropriate model for family medicine. *Earn Med* 1986; **18**: 369–374.

[11] Howie JGR. Research in general practice: pursuit of knowledge or defence of wisdom? *Br Med J* 1984; **289**: 1770–1772.

[12] Malterud K. Illness and disease in female patients. *Scand J Prim Health Care* 1987; **5**: 211–216.

[13] Arborelius A, Bremberg S, Timpka T. What is going on when the general practitioners doesn't grasp the situation? *Fam Prac* 1991; **8**: 3–9.

[14] Mattson B, Winnberg Almqvist E. Attitudes towards predictive testing in Huntingdon's Disease—a deep interview study in Sweden. *Fam Pract* 1991; **8**: 23–27.

[15] Cronbach U. Issues in planning evaluations, in Cronbach U (ed). *Designing Evaluations of Educational and Social Programs.* San Francisco: Jossey Bass, 1982.

[16] Bryman A. *Quantity and Quality in Social Research;* London: Unwin Hyman, 1988.

[17] Von Wright GH. Two traditions, in *Explanation and Understanding.* London: Routledge and Kegan Paul, 1971.

[18] Cochrane AL. *Effectiveness and Efficiency: Random Reflections on Health Services.* Nuffield Provincial Hospitals Trust, 1971.

[19] Dudley RAF. The controlled clinical trial and the advance of reliable knowledge: an outsider looks in. *Br Med J* 1983; **287**: 957–960.

[20] Freer CB. Epidemiology and family medicine. *J Fam Pract* 1979; **8**: 865–866.

[21] Bruusgaard D (ed). *Allmennedisinke Skrifter om Kvalitative Metoder.* Allmenvetenskaplige forskningsradet, Oslo, 1988.

[22] Murphy R, Torrance H (eds). *Evaluating Education: Issues and Methods.* London: Harper and Row, 1987.

[23] Hammersley M, Atkinson P. *Ethnography Principles in Practice.* London: Tavistock, 1983.

[24] Silverman D. *Qualitative Methodology and Sociology.* Aldershot: Gower, 1985.

[25] Schatzmann L, Strauss AL. *Field Research: Strategies for a natural sociology.* Englewood Cliffs, N.J.: Prentice Hall, 1973.

[26] Duffy ME. Designing nursing research: the qualitative-quantitative debate. *J Adv Nurs;* **10**: 225–232.

[27] Nisbet J. Educational Research: The state of the art. In Dockrell WD, Hamilton D (eds) *Rethinking Educational Research.* Princeton Book Co., 1980.

[28] Lessnoff M. *The structure of Social Science: a Philosophical Introduction.* London: George Allen and Unwin, 1974.

[29] Shyrock R. *The Development of Modern Medicine.* University of Wisconsin Press, 1979. First edition, 1936.

[30] Douglas J. *Creative Interviewing.* Sage, 1985.

[31] Glaser B, Strauss A. *The Discovery of Grounded Theory.* Chicago: ldine, 1967.

[32] Coulter A, Noone A, Goldacre M. General practitioners' referrals to specialist outpatient clinics. *Br Med J* **299**: 304–308.

[33] Cronbach LJ. Beyond the two disciplines of scientific psychology, *Am Psychol* **30**: 116–127.

[34] Stenhouse L. The study of samples and the study of cases. *Br Educ Res* **6**: 1–6.

[35] Cornwell J. *Hard-earned Lives.* London: Tavistock, 1984.

[36] Kierkegaard S. *Either/or/.* Edited and translated by Hong HV and Hong EH. Princeton Princeton: University Press, 1987.

COMPETING PARADIGMS IN QUALITATIVE RESEARCH

Chapter 6, Handbook of Qualitative Research. Eds Denzin, N. Lincoln, Y. Ca: Sage, 1994

Egon G. Guba
Yvonna S. Lincoln

AUTHORS' NOTE: We are grateful to Henry Giroux and Robert Stake for their very helpful critiques of an earlier draft of this chapter.

In this chapter we analyze four paradigms that currently are competing, or have until recently competed, for acceptance as the paradigm of choice in informing and guiding inquiry, especially qualitative inquiry: positivism, postpositivism, critical theory and related ideological positions, and constructivism. We acknowledge at once our own commitment to constructivism (which we earlier called "naturalistic inquiry"; Lincoln & Guba, l985); the reader may wish to take that fact into account in judging the appropriateness and usefulness of our analysis.

Although the title of this volume, *Handbook of Qualitative Research*, implies that the term qualitative is an umbrella term superior to the term *paradigm* (and, indeed, that usage is not uncommon), it is our position that it is a term that ought to be reserved for a description of types of methods. From our perspective, both qualitative and quantitative methods may be used appropriately with any research paradigm. Questions of method are secondary to questions of paradigm, which we define as the basic belief system or worldview that guides the investigator, not only in choices of method but in ontologically and epistemologically fundamental ways.

It is certainly the case that interest in alternative paradigms has been stimulated by a growing dissatisfaction with the patent overemphasis on quantitative methods. But as efforts were made to build a case for a renewed interest in qualitative approaches, it became clear that the metaphysical assumptions undergirding the conventional paradigm (the "received view") must be seriously questioned. Thus the emphasis of this chapter is on paradigms, their assumptions. and the implications of those assumptions for a variety of research issues, not on the relative utility of qualitative versus quantitative methods. Nevertheless, as discussions of paradigms/methods over the past decade have often begun with a consideration of problems associated with overquantification, we will also begin there, shifting only later to our predominant interest.

THE QUANTITATIVE/QUALITATIVE DISTINCTION

Historically, there has been a heavy emphasis on quantification in science. Mathematics is often termed the "queen of sciences," and those sciences, such as physics and chemistry, that lend themselves especially well to quantification are generally known as "hard."

Less quantifiable arenas, such as biology (although that is rapidly changing) and particularly the social sciences, are referred to as "soft," less with pejorative intent than to signal their (putative) imprecision and lack of dependability. Scientific maturity is commonly believed to emerge as the degree of quantification found within a given field increases.

That this is the case is hardly surprising. The "received view" of science (positivism, transformed over the course of this century into postpositivism; see below) focuses on efforts to verify (positivism) or falsify (postpositivism) a priori hypotheses, most usefully stated as mathematical (quantitative) propositions or propositions that can be easily converted into precise mathematical formulas expressing functional relationships. Formulaic precision has enormous utility when the aim of science is the prediction and control of natural phenomena. Further, there is already available a powerful array of statistical and mathematical models. Finally, there exists a widespread conviction that only quantitative data are ultimately valid, or of high quality (Sechrest, 1992).

John Stuart Mill (1843/1906) is said to have been the first to urge social scientists to emulate their older, "harder" cousins, promising that if his advice were followed, rapid maturation of these fields, as well as their emancipation from the philosophical and theological strictures that limited them, would follow. Social scientists took this counsel to heart (probably to a degree that would greatly surprise Mill if he were alive today) for other reasons as well. They were the "new kids on the block"; if quantification could lead to the fulfillment of Mill's promise, status and political leverage would accrue that would enormously profit the new practitioners. Imitation might thus lead both to greater acceptance and to more valid knowledge.

CRITIQUES OF THE RECEIVED VIEW

In recent years, however, strong counterpressures against quantification have emerged. Two critiques, one internal to the conventional paradigm (that is, in terms of those metaphysical assumptions that define the nature of positivist inquiry) and one external to it (that is, in terms of those assumptions defining alternative paradigms), have been mounted that seem not only to warrant a reconsideration of the utility of qualitative data but to question the very assumptions on which the putative superiority of quantification has been based.

Internal (Intraparadigm) Critiques

A variety of implicit problems have surfaced to challenge conventional wisdom; several of these are described below.
Context stripping. Precise quantitative approaches that focus on selected subsets of variables necessarily "strip" from consideration, through appropriate controls or randomization, other variables that exist in the context that might, if allowed to exert their effects, greatly alter findings. Further, such exclusionary designs, while increasing the theoretical rigor of a study, detract from its *relevance*, that is, its applicability or generalizability, because their outcomes can be properly applied only in other similarly truncated or contextually stripped situations (another laboratory, for example). Qualitative data, it is argued, can redress that imbalance by providing contextual information.
Exclusion of meaning and purpose. Human behavior, unlike that of physical objects, cannot be understood without reference to the meanings and purposes attached by human actors to their activities. Qualitative data, it is asserted, can provide rich insight into human behavior.
Disjunction of grand theories with local contexts: The etic/emic dilemma. The etic (outsider) theory brought to bear on an inquiry by an investigator (or the hypotheses proposed to be tested) may have little or no meaning within the emic (insider) view of studied individuals, groups, societies, or cultures. Qualitative data, it is affirmed, are useful for uncovering emic views; theories, to be valid, should be qualitatively grounded (Glaser & Strauss, 1967; Strauss & Corbin, 1990). Such grounding is particularly crucial in view of the mounting criticism of social science as failing to provide adequate accounts of nonmainstream lives (the "other") or to provide the material for a criticism of our own Western culture (Marcus & Fischer, 1986).
Inapplicability of general data to individual cases. This problem is sometimes described as the nomothetic/idiographic disjunction. Generalizations, although perhaps statistically meaningful, have no applicability in the individual case (the fact, say, that 80% of individuals presenting given symptoms have lung cancer is at best incomplete evidence that a particular patient presenting with such symptoms has lung cancer). Qualitative data, it is held, can help to avoid such ambiguities.
Exclusion of the discovery dimension in inquiry. Conventional emphasis on the verification of specific, a priori hypotheses glosses over the source of those hypotheses, usually arrived at by what is commonly termed the discovery process. In the received view only empirical inquiry deserves to be called "science." Quantitative normative methodology is thus privileged over the insights of creative and divergent thinkers. The call for qualitative inputs is expected to redress this imbalance.

External (Extraparadigm) Critiques

The intraparadigm problems noted above offer a weighty challenge to conventional methodology, but could be eliminated, or at least ameliorated, by greater use of qualitative data. Many critics of the received view are content to stop at that point; hence many of the calls for more qualitative inputs have been limited to this methods-level accommodation. But an even weightier challenge has been mounted by critics who have proposed *alternative paradigms* that involve not only qualification of approaches but fundamental adjustments in the basic assumptions that guide inquiry altogether. Their rejection of the received view can be justified on a number of grounds (Bernstein, 1988; Guba, 1990; Ilesse, 1980; Lincoln & Cuba, 1985; Reason & Rowan, 1981), but chief among them are the following.[1]
The theory-ladenness of facts. Conventional approaches to research involving the verification or falsification of hypotheses assume the independence of theoretical and observational languages. If an inquiry is to be objective, hypotheses must be stated in ways that are independent of the way in which the facts needed to test them are collected. But it now seems established beyond objection that theories and facts are quite *interdependent* – that is, that facts are facts only within some theoretical framework. Thus a fundamental assumption of the received view is exposed as dubious. If hypotheses and observations are not independent, "facts" can be viewed only through a theoretical "window" and objectivity is undermined.
The underdetermination of theory. This problem is also known as the problem of induction. Not only are facts determined by the theory window through which one looks for them, but different theory windows might be equally well supported by the same set of "facts." Although it may be possible, given a coherent theory, to derive by deduction what facts ought to exist, it is never possible, given a coherent set of facts, to arrive by *induction* at a single, ineluctable theory. Indeed, it is this difficulty that led philosophers such as Popper (1968) to reject the notion of theory *verification* in favor of the notion of theory *falsification*. Whereas a million white swans can never establish, with complete confidence, the proposition that all swans are white, one black swan can completely falsify it. The historical position of science that it can, by its methods, ultimately converge on the "rear" truth is thus brought sharply into question.
The value-ladenness of facts. Just as theories and facts are not independent, neither are values and facts. Indeed, it can be argued that theories are themselves value statements. Thus putative "facts" are viewed not only through a theory window but through a value window as well. The value-free posture of the received view is compromised.
The interactive nature of the inquirer-inquired into dyad. The received view of science pictures the inquirer as standing behind a one-way mirror, viewing natural phenomena as they happen and recording them objectively. The inquirer (when using proper methodology) does not influence the phenomena or vice versa. But evidence such as the Heisenberg uncertainty principle and the Bohr complementarity

principle have shattered that ideal in the hard sciences (Lincoln & Guba, 1985); even greater skepticism must exist for the social sciences. Indeed, the notion that findings are created through the interaction of inquirer and phenomenon (which, in the social sciences, is usually people) is often a more plausible description of the inquiry process than is the notion that findings are discovered through objective observation "as they *really* are, and as they *really* work."

The intraparadigm critiques, although exposing many inherent problems in the received view and, indeed, proposing some useful responses to them, are nevertheless of much less interest or weight – than the extraparadigm critiques, which raise problems of such consequence that the received view is being widely questioned. Several alternative paradigms have been proposed, some of which rest on quite unconventional assumptions. It is useful, therefore, to inquire about the nature of paradigms and what it is that distinguishes one inquiry paradigm from another.

THE NATURE OF PARADIGMS

Paradigms as Basic Belief Systems Based on Ontological, Epistemological, and Methodological Assumptions

A paradigm may be viewed as a set of *basic beliefs* (or metaphysics) that deals with ultimates or first principles. It represents a worldview that defines, for its holder, the nature of the "world," the individual's place in it, and the range of possible relationships to that world and its parts, as, for example, cosmologies and theologies do.[2] The beliefs are basic in the sense that they must be accepted simply on faith (however well argued); there is no way to establish their ultimate truthfulness. If there were, the philosophical debates reflected in these pages would have been resolved millennia ago.

Inquiry paradigms define for *inquirers* what it is they are about, and what falls within and outside the limits of legitimate inquiry. The basic beliefs that define inquiry paradigms can be summarized by the responses given by proponents of any given paradigm to three fundamental questions, which are interconnected in such a way that the answer given to any one question, taken in any order, constrains how the others may be answered. We have selected an order that we believe reflects a logical (if not necessary) primacy:

1. *The ontological question.* What is the form and nature of reality and, therefore, what is there that can be known about it? For example, if a "real" world is assumed, then what can be known about it is "how things really are" and "how things really work." Then only those questions that relate to matters of "real" existence and "real" action are admissible; other questions, such as those concerning matters of aesthetic or moral significance, fall outside the realm of legitimate scientific inquiry.

2. *The epistemological question.* What is the nature of the relationship between the knower or would-be knower and what can be known? The answer that can be given to this question is constrained by the answer already given to the ontological question; that is, not just any relationship can now be postulated. So if, for example, a "real" reality is assumed, then the posture of the knower must be one of objective detachment or value freedom in order to be able to discover "how things really are" and "how things really work." (Conversely, assumption of an objectivist posture implies the existence of a "real" world to be objective about.)

3. *The methodological question.* How can the inquirer (would-be knower) go about finding out whatever he or she believes can be known? Again, the answer that can be given to this question is constrained by answers already given to the first two questions; that is, not just any methodology is appropriate. For example, a "real" reality pursued by an "objective" inquirer mandates control of possible confounding factors, whether the methods are qualitative (say, observational) or quantitative (say, analysis of covariance). (Conversely, selection of a manipulative methodology-the experiment, say-implies the ability to be objective and a real world to be objective about.) The methodological question cannot be reduced to a question of methods; methods must be fitted to a predetermined methodology.

These three questions serve as the major foci around which we will analyze each of the four paradigms to be considered.

Paradigms as Human Constructions

We have already noted that paradigms. as sets of basic beliefs, are not open to proof in any conventional sense; there is no way to elevate one over another on the basis of ultimate, foundational criteria. (We should note, however, that that state of affairs does not doom us to a radical relativist posture; see Cuba, 1992.) In our opinion, any given paradigm represents simply the most informed and sophisticated view that its proponents have been able to devise, given the way they have chosen to respond to the three defining questions. And, we argue, the sets of answers given are in *all* cases *human constructions*; that is, they are all inventions of the human mind and hence subject to human error. No construction is or can be incontrovertibly right; advocates of any particular construction must rely on *persuasiveness* and *utility* rather than *proof* in arguing their position.

What is true of paradigms is true of our analyses as well. Everything that we shall say subsequently is *also* a human construction: ours. The reader cannot be compelled to accept our analyses, or our arguments, on the basis of incontestable logic or indisputable evidence; we can only hope to be persuasive and to demonstrate the utility of our position for, say, the public policy arena (Guba & Lincoln, 1989; House, 1977). We do ask the reader to suspend his or her disbelief until our argument is complete and can be judged as a whole.

The Basic Beliefs of Received and Alternative Inquiry Paradigms

We begin our analysis with descriptions of the responses that we believe proponents of each paradigm would make to the three questions outlined above. These responses (as constructed by us) are displayed in Table 6.1, which consists of three rows corresponding to the ontological, epistemological, and methodological questions, and four columns corresponding to the four paradigms to be discussed. The term *positivism* denotes the "received view" that has dominated the formal discourse in the physical and social sciences for some 400 years, whereas *postpositivism* represents efforts of the past few decades to respond in a limited way (that is, while remaining within essentially the same set of basic beliefs) to the most problematic criticisms of positivism. The term *critical theory* is (for us) a blanket term denoting a set of several alternative paradigms, including additionally (but not limited to) neo-Marxism, feminism, materialism, and participatory inquiry. Indeed, critical theory may itself usefully be divided into three substrands: poststructuralism, postmodernism, and a blending of these two. Whatever their differences, the common breakaway assumption of all these variants is that of the value-determined nature of inquiry – an epistemological difference. Our grouping of these positions into a single category is a judgment call; we will not try to do justice to the individual points of view. The term *constructivism* denotes an alternative paradigm whose breakaway assumption is the move from ontological realism to ontological relativism. These positions will become clear in the subsequent exposition.

Two important caveats need to be mentioned. First, although we are inclined to believe that the paradigms we are about to describe can have meaning even in the realm of the physical sciences, we will not defend that belief here. Accordingly, our subsequent comments should be understood to be limited to the *social sciences* only. Second, we note that except for positivism, the paradigms discussed are all still in formative stages; no final agreements have been reached even among their proponents about their definitions, meanings, or implications. Thus our discussion should be considered tentative and subject to further revision and reformulation.

We will first look down the columns of Table 6.1 to illustrate the positions of each paradigm with respect to the three questions, following with a look across rows to compare and contrast the positions of the paradigms.[3] Limitations of space make it impossible for us to develop our assertions in any depth. The reader will be able to find other evidence, pro and con, in other chapters of this volume, particularly in Chapters 7-11.

Intraparadigm Analyses (Columns of Table 6.1)

Column I: Positivism
Ontology: realism (commonly called "naive realism"). An apprehendable reality is assumed to exist, driven by immutable natural laws and mechanisms. Knowledge of the "way things are" is conventionally summarized in the form of time- and context-free generalizations, some of which take the form of cause-effect laws. Research can, in principle, converge on the "true" state of affairs. The

Table 6.1
Basic Beliefs (Metaphysics) of Alternative Inquiry Paradigms

Item	Positivism	Postpositivism	Critical Theory et aL	Constructivism
Ontology	naive realis "real" reality but apprehendable	critical realism- "real" reality but only imperfectly and probabilistically apprehendable	historical realism- virtual reality shaped by social. political. cultural. economic. ethnic, and gender values; crystallized over time	relativisloeal and specific constructed realities
Epistemology	dualist'objectivist; findings true	modified dualist! objectivist; critical tradition'community; findings probably true	transactional! subjectivist; value- mediated findings	transactional! subjectivist; created findings
Methodology	experimental/ manipulative; verification of hypotheses; chiefly quantitative methods	modified experi- mentalimanipulative; critical multiplism; falsification of hypotheses; may include qualitative methods	dialogicdialectical	hermeneutical!dialeetical

basic posture of the paradigm is argued to be both reductionist and deterministic (Hesse. 1980).

Epistemology: Dualist and objectivist. The investigator and the investigated "object" are assumed to be independent entities, and the investigator to be capable of studying the object without influencing it or being influenced by it. When influence in either direction (threats to validity) is recognized, or even suspected, various strategies are followed to reduce or eliminate it. Inquiry takes place as through a one-way mirror. Values and biases are prevented from influencing outcomes, so long as the prescribed procedures are rigorously followed. Replicable findings are, in fact, "true."

Methodology: Experimental and manipulative. Questions and/or hypotheses are stated in propositional form and subjected to empirical test to verify them; possible confounding conditions must be carefully controlled (manipulated) to prevent outcomes from being improperly influenced.

Column 2: Postpositivism

Ontology: Critical realism. Reality is assumed to exist but to be only imperfectly apprehendable because of basically flawed human intellectual mechanisms and the fundamentally intractable nature of phenomena. The ontology is labeled as critical realism (Cook & Campbell, 1979) because of the posture of proponents that claims about reality must be subjected to the widest possible critical examination to facilitate apprehending reality as closely as possible (but never perfectly).

Epistemology: Modified dualist/objectivist. Dualism is largely abandoned as not possible to maintain, but objectivity remains a "regulatory ideal"; special emphasis is placed on external "guardians" of objectivity such as critical traditions (Do the findings "fit" with pre-existing knowledge?) and the critical community (such as editors, referees, and professional peers). Replicated findings are probably true (but always subject to falsification).

Methodology: Modified experimental/manipulative. Emphasis is placed on "critical multiplism" (a refurbished version of triangulation) as a way of falsifying (rather than verifying) hypotheses. The methodology aims to redress some of the problems noted above (intraparadigm critiques) by doing inquiry in more natural settings, collecting more situational information, and reintroducing discovery as an element in inquiry, and, in the social sciences particularly, soliciting emic viewpoints to assist in determining the meanings and purposes that people ascribe to their actions, as well as to contribute to "grounded theory" (Glaser & Strauss, 1967; Strauss & Corbin, 1990). All these aims are accomplished largely through the increased utilization of qualitative techniques.

Column 3: Critical Theory and Related Ideological Positions

Ontology: Historical realism. A reality is assumed to be apprehendable that was once plastic, but that was, over time, shaped by a congeries of social, political, cultural, economic, ethnic, and gender factors, and then crystallized (reified) into a series of structures that are now (inappropriately) taken as "real," that is, natural and immutable. For all practical purposes the structures are "real," a virtual or historical reality.

Epistemology: Transactional and subjectivist. The investigator and the investigated object are assumed to be interactively linked, with the values of the investigator (and of situated "others") inevitably influencing the inquiry. Findings are therefore *value mediated*. Note that this posture effectively challenges the traditional distinction between ontology and epistemology; what can be known is inextricably intertwined with the interaction between a *particular* investigator and a *particular* object or group. The dashed line separating the ontological and epistemological rows of Table 6.1 is intended to reflect this fusion.

Methodology: Dialogic and dialectical. The transactional nature of inquiry requires a dialogue between the investigator and the subjects of the inquiry; that dialogue must be dialectical in nature to transform ignorance and misapprehensions (accepting historically mediated structures as immutable) into more informed consciousness (seeing how the structures might be changed and comprehending the actions required to effect change), or, as Giroux (1988) puts it, "as transformative intellectuals, . . . to uncover and excavate those forms of historical and subjugated knowledges that point to experiences of suffering, conflict, and collective struggle; . . . to link the notion of historical undestanding to elements of critique and hope" (p. 213). Transformational inquirers demonstrate "transformational leadership" (Burns, 1978). (For more discussion of critical theory, see the contributions in this volume by Olesen, Chapter 9; Stanfield, Chapter 10; and Kincheloe & McLaren, Chapter 8.)

Column 4: Constructivism

Ontology: Relativist. Realities are apprehendable in the form of multiple, intangible mental constructions, socially and experientially based, local and specific in nature (although elements are often shared among many individuals and even across cultures), and dependent for their form and content on the individual persons or groups holding the constructions. Constructions are not more or less "true," in any absolute sense, but simply more or less informed and/or sophisticated. Constructions are alterable, as are their associated "realities." This position should be distinguished from both nominalism and idealism (see Reese, 1980, for an explication of these several ideas).

Epistemology: Transactional and subjectivist. The investigator and the object of investigation are assumed to be interactively linked so that the "findings" are *literally created* as the investigation proceeds. The conventional distinction between ontology and epistemology disappears, as in the case of critical theory. Again, the dashed line of Table 6.1 reflects this fact. *Methodology: Hermeneutical and dialectical.* The variable and personal (intramental) nature of social constructions suggests that individual constructions can be elicited and refined only through interaction *between* and *among* investigator and respondents. These varying constructions are interpreted using conventional hermeneutical techniques, and are compared and contrasted through a dialectical interchange. The final aim is to distill a consensus construction that is more informed and sophisticated than any of the predecessor constructions (including, of course, the etic construction of the investigator). (For more about constructivism, see also Schwandt, Chapter 7, this volume.)

CROSS-PARADIGM ANALYSES (ROWS OF TABLE 6.1)

Having noted briefly the positions that proponents of each paradigm might take with respect to the three paradigm-defining questions, it is useful to look across rows to compare and contrast those positions among the several paradigms.

Ontology

Moving from left to right across Table 6.1, we note the move from

1. positivism's position of naive realism, assuming an objective external reality upon which inquiry can converge; to
2. postpositivism's critical realism, which still assumes an objective reality but grants that it can be apprehended only imperfectly and probabilistically; to
3. critical theory's historical realism, which assumes an apprehendable reality consisting of historically situated structures that are, in the absence of insight, as limiting and confining as if they were real; to
4. constructivism's relativism, which assumes multiple, apprehendable, and sometimes conflicting social realities that are the products of human intellects, but that may change as their constructors become more informed and sophisticated.

It is the ontological position that most differentiates constructivism from the other three paradigms.

Epistemology

We note the move from
1. positivism's dualist, objectivist assumption that enables the investigator to determine "how things really are" and "how things really work"; to
2. postpositivism's modified dualist/objectivist assumption that it is possible to approximate (but never fully know) reality; to
3. critical theory's transactional/subjectivist assumption that knowledge is value mediated and hence value dependent; to
4. constructivism's somewhat similar but broader transactional/subjectivist assumption that sees

knowledge as created in interaction among investigator and respondents.

It is their epistemological positions that most differentiate critical theory and constructivism from the other two paradigms.

Methodology

We note the move from
1. positivism's experimental/manipulative methodology that focuses on verification of hypotheses; to
2. postpositivism's modified experimental/manipulative methodology invested in critical multiplism focusing on falsification of hypotheses; to
3. critical theory's *dialogic/dialectical* methodology aimed at the reconstruction of previously held constructions; to
4. constructivism's hermeneutic/dialectic methodology aimed at the reconstruction of previously held constructions.

IMPLICATIONS OF EACH PARADIGM'S POSITION ON SELECTED PRACTICAL ISSUES (ROWS OF TABLE 6.2)

Differences in paradigm assumptions cannot be dismissed as mere "philosophical" differences; implicitly or explicitly, these positions have important consequences for the practical conduct of inquiry, as well as for the interpretation of findings and policy choices. We have elected to discuss these consequences for ten salient issues.

The entries in Table 6.2, which consists of four columns corresponding to the four paradigms and ten rows corresponding to the ten issues, summarize our interpretation of the major implications. The reader will note that the first four issues (inquiry aim, nature of knowledge, knowledge accumulation, and quality criteria) are among those deemed especially important by positivists and postpositivists; they are therefore the issues on which alternative paradigms are most frequently attacked. The fifth and sixth (values and ethics) are issues taken seriously by all paradigms, although conventional and emergent responses are quite different. Finally, the last four issues (voice, training, accommodation, and hegemony) are those deemed especially important by alternative proponents; they represent areas on which the received view is considered particularly vulnerable. The entries in the table are based only in part on public positions, given that not all issues have been addressed by all paradigms' proponents. In some cases, therefore, we have supplied entries that we believe follow logically from the basic metaphysical (ontological, epistemological, and methodological) postures of the paradigms. To take one example, the issue of voice is rarely addressed directly by positivists or postpositivists, but we believe the entry "disinterested scientist" is one that would be given by those proponents were they to be challenged on this matter.

Table 6.2

Paradigm Positions on Selected Practical Issues

Issue	Positivism	Postpositivism	Critical Theory *et al.*	Constructivism
Inquiry aim	explanation: prediction and control		critique and transformation; restitution and emancipation	understanding; reconstruction
Nature of knowledge	verified hypotheses established as facts or laws	nonfalsified hypotheses that are probable facts or laws	structural/historical insights	individual reconstructions coalescing around consensus
Knowledge accumulation	accretion – "building clocks" adding to "edifice of knowledge"; generalizations and cause-effect linkages		historical revisionism; generalization by similarity	more informed and sophisticated reconstructions; vicarious experience
Goodness or quality criteria	conventional benchmarks of "rigor": internal and external validity, reliability, and objectivity		historical situatedness; erosion of ignorance; action stimulus	trustworthiness and authenticity and misapprehensions;
Values	excluded – influence denied		included – formative	
Ethics	extrinsic; tilt toward deception		intrinsic; moral tilt toward revelation	intrinsic; process tilt toward revelation; special problems
Voice	"disinterested scientist" as informer of decision makers, policy makers, and change agents		"transformative intellectual" as advocate and activist	"passionate participant" as facilitator of multi-voice reconstruction
Training	technical and quantitative; substantive theories	technical; quantitative and qualitative; substantive theories	resocialization; qualitative and quantitative; history; values of altruism and empowerment	
Accommodation	commensurable		incommensurable	
Hegemony	in control of publication, funding. promotion. and tenure		seeking recognition and input	

An immediately apparent difference between Table 6.1 and Table 6.2 is that whereas in the former case it was possible to make a distinct entry for every cell, in the case of Table 6.2 there is considerable overlap within rows, particularly for the positivist and postpositivist columns. Indeed, even for those issues in which the entries in those two columns are different, the differences appear to be minor. In contrast, one may note the major differences found between these two paradigms and the critical theory and constructivist paradigms, which tend also to differ among themselves.

We have formulated the issues as questions, which follow.

Row 1: What is the aim or purpose of inquiry?
Positivism and postpositivism. For both these paradigms the aim of inquiry is *explanation* (von Wright, 1971), ultimately enabling the *prediction* and control of phenomena, whether physical or human. As Hesse (1930) has suggested, the ultimate criterion for progress in these paradigms is that the capability of "scientists" to predict and control should improve over time. The reductionism and determinism implied by this position should be noted. The inquirer is cast in the role of "expert," a situation that seems to award special, perhaps even unmerited, privilege to the investigator. *Critical theory.* The aim of inquiry is the *critique and*

transformation of the social, political, cultural, economic, ethnic, and gender structures that constrain and exploit humankind, by engagement in confrontation, even conflict. The criterion for progress is that over time, restitution and emancipation should occur and persist. Advocacy and activism are key concepts. The inquirer is cast in the role of instigator and facilitator, implying that the inquirer understands a priori what transformations are needed. But we should note that some of the more radical stances in the criticalist camp hold that judgment about needed transformations should be reserved to those whose lives are most affected by transformations: the inquiry participants themselves (Lincoln, in press).

Constructivism. The aim of inquiry is *understanding and reconstruction* of the constructions that people (including the inquirer) initially hold, aiming toward consensus but still open to new interpretations as information and sophistication improve. The criterion for progress is that over time, everyone formulates more informed and sophisticated constructions and becomes more aware of the content and meaning of competing constructions. Advocacy and activism are also key concepts is this view. The inquirer is cast in the role of participant and facilitator in this process, a position that some critics have faulted on the grounds that it expands the inquirer's role beyond reasonable expectations of expertise and competence (Carr & Kemmis, 1986).

Row 2: What is the nature of knowledge?

Positivism. Knowledge consists of verified hypotheses that can be accepted as facts or laws.

Postpositivism. Knowledge consists of nonfalsified hypotheses that can be regarded as probable facts or laws.

Critical theory. Knowledge consists of a series of structural/historical insights that will be transformed as time passes. Transformations occur when ignorance and misapprehensions give way to more informed insights by means of a dialectical interaction.

Constructivism. Knowledge consists of those constructions about which there is relative consensus (or at least some movement toward consensus) among those competent (and, in the case of more arcane material, trusted) to interpret the substance of the construction. Multiple "knowledges" can coexist when equally competent (or trusted) interpreters disagree, and/or depending on social, political, cultural, economic, ethnic, and gender factors that differentiate the interpreters. These constructions are subject to continuous revision, with changes most likely to occur when relatively different constructions are brought into juxtaposition in a dialectical context.

Row 3: How does knowledge accumulate?

Positivism and postpositivism. Knowledge accumulates by a process of accretion, with each fact (or probable fact) serving as a kind of building block that, when placed into its proper niche, adds to the growing "edifice of knowledge." When the facts take the form of generalizations or cause-effect linkages, they may be used most efficiently for prediction and control. Generalizations may then be made, with predictable confidence, to a population of settings.

Critical theory. Knowledge does not accumulate in an absolute sense; rather, it grows and changes through a dialectical process of historical revision that continuously erodes ignorance and misapprehensions and enlarges more informed insights. Generalization can occur when the mix of social, political, cultural, economic, ethnic, and gender circumstances and values is similar across settings.

Constructivism. Knowledge accumulates only in a relative sense through the formation of ever more informed and sophisticated constructions via the hermeneutical/dialectical process, as varying constructions are brought into juxtaposition. One important mechanism for transfer of knowledge from one setting to another is the provision of vicarious experience, often supplied by case study reports (see Stake, Chapter 14, this volume).

Row 4: What criteria are appropriate for judging the goodness or quality of an inquiry?

Positivism and postpositivism. The appropriate criteria are the conventional benchmarks of "rigor": internal validity (isomorphism of findings with reality), external validity (generalizability), reliability (in the sense of stability), and objectivity (distanced and neutral observer). These criteria depend on the realist ontological position; without the assumption, isomorphisin of findings with reality can have no meaning, strict generalizability to a parent population is impossible, stability cannot be assessed for inquiry into a phenomenon if the phenomenon itself can change, and objectivity cannot be achieved because there is nothing from which one can be "distant."

Critical theory. The appropriate criteria are historical situatedness of the inquiry (i.e., that it takes account of the social, political, cultural, economic, ethnic, and gender antecedents of the studied situation), the extent to which the inquiry acts to erode ignorance and misapprehensions, and the extent to which it provides a stimulus to action, that is, to the transformation of the existing structure.

Constructivism. Two sets of criteria have been proposed: the *trustworthiness* criteria of credibility (paralleling internal validity), transferability (paralleling external validity), dependability (paralleling reliability), and confirmability (paralleling objectivity) (Guba, 1981; Lincoln & Guba, 1985); and the *authenticity* criteria of fairness, ontological authenticity (enlarges personal constructions), educative authenticity (leads to improved understanding of constructions of others), catalytic authenticity (stimulates to action), and tactical authenticity (empowers action) (Guba & Lincoln, 1989). The former set represents an early effort to resolve the quality issue for constructivism; although these criteria have been well received, their parallelism to positivist criteria makes them suspect. The latter set overlaps to some extent those of critical theory but goes beyond them, particularly the two of ontological authenticity and educative authenticity. The issue of quality criteria in constructivism is nevertheless not well resolved, and further critique is needed.

Row 5: What is the role of values in inquiry?
Positivism and postpositivism. In both these paradigms values are specifically excluded; indeed, the paradigm is claimed to be "value free" by virtue of its epistemological posture. Values are seen as confounding variables that cannot be allowed a role in a putatively objective inquiry (even when objectivity is, in the case of postpositivism, but a regulatory ideal).
Critical theory and constructivism. In both these paradigms values have pride of place; they are seen as ineluctable in shaping (in the case of constructivism, creating) inquiry outcomes. Furthermore, even if it were possible, excluding values would not be countenanced. To do so would be inimical to the interests of the powerless and of "at-risk" audiences, whose original (emic) constructions deserve equal consideration with those of other, more powerful audiences and of the inquirer (etic). Constructivism, which sees the inquirer as orchestrator and facilitator of the inquiry process, is more likely to stress this point than is critical theory, which tends to cast the inquirer in a more authoritative role.

Row 6: What is the place of ethics in inquiry?
Positivism and postpositivism. In both these paradigms ethics is an important consideration, and it is taken very seriously by inquirers, but it is *extrinsic* to the inquiry process itself. Hence ethical behavior is formally policed by *external* mechanisms, such as professional codes of conduct and human subjects committees. Further, the realist ontology undergirding these paradigms provides a tilt toward the use of deception, which, it is argued in certain cases, is warranted to determine how "things *really* are and work" or for the sake of some "higher social good" or some "clearer truth" (Bok, 1978, 1982; Diener & Crandall, 1978).
Critical theory. Ethics is more nearly *intrinsic* to this paradigm, as implied by the intent to erode ignorance and misapprehensions, and to take full account of values and historical situatedness in the inquiry process. Thus there is a moral tilt that the inquirer be revelatory (in the rigorous meaning of "fully informed consent") rather than deceptive. Of course, these considerations do not *prevent* unethical behavior, but they do provide some process barriers that make it more difficult.
Constructivism. Ethics is *intrinsic* to this paradigm also because of the inclusion of participant values in the inquiry (starting with respondents' existing constructions and working toward increased information and sophistication in their constructions as well as in the inquirer's construction). There is an incentive – a *process tilt* – for revelation; hiding the inquirer's intent is destructive of the aim of uncovering and improving constructions. In addition, the

hermeneutical/dialectical methodology itself provides a strong but not infallible safeguard against deception. However, the close personal interactions required by the methodology may produce special and often sticky problems of confidentiality and anonymity, as well as other interpersonal difficulties (Guba & Lincoln, 1989).

Row 7: What voice is mirrored in the inquirer's activities, especially those directed at change?
Positivism and postpositivism. The inquirer's voice is that of the "disinterested scientist" informing decision makers, policy makers, and change agents, who independently use this scientific information, at least in part, to form, explain, and justify actions, policies, and change proposals.
Critical theory. The inquirer's voice is that of the "transformative intellectual" (Giroux, 1988) who has expanded consciousness and so is in a position to confront ignorance and misapprehensions. Change is facilitated as individuals develop greater insight into the existing state of affairs (the nature and extent of their exploitation) and are stimulated to act on it.
Constructivism. The inquirer's voice is that of the "passionate participant" (Lincoln, 1991) actively engaged in facilitating the "multi voice" reconstruction of his or her own construction as well as those of all other participants. Change is facilitated as reconstructions are formed and individuals are stimulated to act on them.

Row 8: What are the implications of each paradigm for the training of novice inquirers?
Positivism. Novices are trained primarily in technical knowledge about measurement, design, and quantitative methods, with less but substantial emphasis on formal theories of the phenomena in their substantive specialties.
Postpositivism. Novices are trained in ways paralleling the positivist mode, but with the addition of qualitative methods, often for the purpose of ameliorating the problems noted in the opening paragraphs of this chapter.
Critical theory and constructivism. Novices must first be resocialized from their early and usually intense exposure to the received view of science. That resocialization cannot be accomplished without thorough schooling in the postures and techniques of positivism and postpositivism. Students must come to appreciate paradigm differences (summarized in Table 6.1) and, in that context, to master both qualitative and quantitative methods. The former are essential because of their role in carrying out the dialogic/dialectical or hermeneutical/dialectical methodologies; the latter because they can play a useful informational role in all paradigms. They must also be helped to understand the social, political, cultural, economic, ethnic, and gender history and structure that serve as the surround for their inquiries, and to incorporate the values of altruism and empowerment in their work.

Row 9: Are these paradigms necessarily in conflict? Is it possible to accommodate these several views within a single conceptual framework?

Positivism and postpositivism. Proponents of these two paradigms, given their foundational orientation, take the position that all paradigms can be accommodated – that is, that there exists, or will be found to exist, some common rational structure to which all questions of difference can be referred for resolution. The posture is reductionist and assumes the possibility of point-by-point comparisons (commensurability), an issue about which there continues to be a great deal of disagreement.

Critical theory and constructivism. Proponents of these two paradigms join in affirming the basic incommensurability of the paradigms (although they would agree that positivism and postpositivism are commensurable, and would probably agree that critical theory and constructivism are commensurable). The basic beliefs of the paradigms are believed to be essentially contradictory. For constructivists, either there is a "real" reality or there is not (although one might wish to resolve this problem differently in considering the physical versus the human realms), and thus constructivism and positivism/postpositivism cannot be logically accommodated anymore than, say, the ideas of flat versus round earth can be logically accommodated. For critical theorists and constructivists, inquiry is either value free or it is not; again, logical accommodation seems impossible. Realism and relativism, value freedom and value boundedness, cannot coexist in any internally consistent metaphysical system, which condition of consistency, it is stipulated, is essentially met by each of the candidate paradigms. Resolution of this dilemma will necessarily await the emergence of a metaparadigm that renders the older, accommodated paradigms not less true, but simply irrelevant.

Row 10: Which of the paradigms exercises hegemony over the others? That is, which is predominantly influential?

Positivism and postpositivism. Proponents of positivism gained hegemony over the past several centuries as earlier Aristotelian and theological paradigms were abandoned. But the mantle of hegemony has in recent decades gradually fallen on the shoulders of the postpositivists, the "natural" heirs of positivism. Postpositivists (and indeed many residual positivists) tend to control publication outlets, funding sources, promotion and tenure mechanisms, dissertation committees, and other sources of power and influence. They were, at least until about 1980, the "in" group, and continue to represent the strongest voice in professional decision making.

Critical theory and constructivism. Proponents of critical theory and constructivism are still seeking recognition and avenues for input. Over the past decade, it has become more and more possible for them to achieve acceptance, as attested by increasing inclusion of relevant papers in journals and professional meetings, the development of new journal outlets, the growing acceptability of "qualitative" dissertations, the inclusion of "qualitative" guidelines by some funding agencies and programs, and the like. But in all likelihood, critical theory and constructivism will continue to play secondary, although important and progressively more influential, roles in the near future.

CONCLUSION

The metaphor of the "paradigm wars" described by Gage (1989) is undoubtedly overdrawn. Describing the discussions and altercations of the past decade or two as wars paints the matter as more confrontational than necessary. A resolution of paradigm differences can occur only when a new paradigm emerges that is more informed and sophisticated than any existing one. That is most likely to occur if and when proponents of these several points of view come together to discuss their differences, not to argue the sanctity of their views. Continuing dialogue among paradigm proponents of all stripes will afford the best avenue for moving toward a responsive and congenial relationship.

We hope that in this chapter we have illustrated the need for such a discussion by clearly delineating the differences that currently exist, and by showing that those differences have significant implications at the practical level. Paradigm issues are crucial; no inquirer, we maintain, ought to go about the business of inquiry without being clear about just what paradigm informs and guides his or her approach.

NOTES

1. Many of the objections listed here were first enunciated by positivists themselves; indeed, we might argue that the postpositivist position represents an attempt to transform positivism in ways that take account of these same objections. The naive positivist position of the sixteenth through the nineteenth centuries is no longer held by anyone even casually acquainted with these problems. Although we would concede that the postpositivist position, as enunciated, for example, by Denis Phillips (1987, 1990a, 1990b), represents a considerable improvement over classic positivism, it fails to make a clean break. It represents a kind of "damage control" rather than a reformulation of basic principles. The notion that these problems required a paradigm shift was poorly recognized until the publication of Thomas Kuhn's landmark work, *The Structure of Scientific Revolutions* (1962, 1970), and even then proceeded but slowly. Nevertheless, the contributions of pre-Kuhnian critics should be recognized and applauded.

2. We are reminded by Robert Stake (personal communication. 1993) that the view of paradigms that we present here should not "exclude a belief that there are worlds within worlds, unending, each with its own paradigms. Infinitesimals have their own cosmologies."

3. It is unlikely that a practitioner of any paradigm

would agree that our summaries closely describe what he or she thinks or does. Workaday scientists rarely have either the time or the inclination to assess what they do in philosophical terms. We do contend, however, that these descriptions are apt as broad brush strokes, if not always at the individual level.

References

Bernstein, R. (1988). *Beyond objectivism and relativism.* Philadelphia: University of Pennsylvania Press.

Bok, S(1978). *Lies: Moral choice in public and private life.* New York: Random House.

Bok, S. (1982). *Secrets: On the ethics of concealment and revelation.* New York: Pantheon.

Burns, J. (1978). *Leadership.* New York: Harper.

Carr, W., & Kemmis, S. (1986). *Becoming critical: Education, knowledge and action research.* London: Falmer.

Cook, T., & Campbell, D. T. (1979). Quasi-experimentation: Design and analysis issues for field settings. Chicago: Rand McNally.

Diener, E., & Crandall, R. (1978). *Ethics in social and behavioral research.* Chicago: University of Chicago Press.

Gage, N. (1989). The paradigm wars and their aftermath: A 'historical' sketch of research and teaching since 1989. *Educational Research, 18,* 4-10.

Giroux, H. (1988). *Schooling and the struggle for public life: Critical pedagogy in the modern age.* Minneapolis: University of Minnesota Press.

Glaser, B. G., & Strauss, A. L. (1967). *The discovery of grounded theory: Strategies for qualitative research.* Chicago: Aldine.

Guba, E.G. (1981). Criteria for assessing the trustworthiness of naturalistic inquiries. *Educational Communication and Technology Journal, 29,* 75-92.

Guba, E. G. (Ed.). (1990). *The paradigm dialog.* Newbury Park, CA: Sage.

Guba, E. G. (1992). Relativism. *Curriculum Inquiry. 22,* 17-24.

Guba, E. G., & Lincoln, Y. S.(1989). *Fourth generation evaluation.* Newbury Park, CA: Sage.

Hesse, E. (1980). *Revolutions and reconstructions in the philosophy of science.* Bloomington: Indiana University Press.

House, E. (1977). *The logic of evaluative argument.* Los Angeles: University of California Center for the Study of Evaluation.

Kuhn, T. S. (1962). *The structure of scientific revolutions.* Chicago: University of Chicago Press.

Kuhn, T. S. (1970). *The structure of scientific revolutions* (2nd ed.). Chicago: University of Chicago Press.

Lincoln, Y. S. (1991). *The detached observer and the passionate participant: Discourses in inquiry and science.* Paper presented at the annual meeting of the American Educational Research Association, Chicago.

Lincoln, Y. S. (in press). I and thou: Method and voice in research with the silenced. In D. McLaughlin & W. Tierney (Eds.), *Naming silenced lives.* New York: Praeger.

Lincoln, Y. S., & Guba, E. G. (1985). *Naturalistic inquiry.* Beverly Hills, CA: Sage.

Marcus, G., & Fischer, M. (1986). *Anthropology as cultural critique: An experimental moment in the human sciences.* Chicago: University of Chicago Press.

Mill, J. S. (1906). *A system of logic.* London: Longmans Green. (Original work published 1843)

Phillips, D. C. (1987). *Philosophy, science, and social inquiry.* Oxford: Pergamon.

Phillips, D. C. (1990a). Postpositivistic science: Myths and realities. In E. G. Guba (Ed.), *The paradigm dialog* (pp. 31-45). Newbury Park, CA: Sage.

Phillips, D. C. (1990b). Subjectivity and objectivity: An objective inquiry. In E. Eisner & A. Peshicin (Eds.), *Qualitative inquiry in education* (pp. 19-37). New York: Teachers College Press.

Popper, K. (1968). *Conjectures and refutations.* New York: Harper & Row.

Reason, P., & Rowan, J. (1981). *Human inquiry.* New York: John Wiley.

Reese, W. (1980). *Dictionary of philosophy and religion.* Atlantic Highlands, NJ: Humanities Press.

Sechrest, L. (1992). Roots: Back to our first generations. *Evaluation Practice, 13,* 1-8.

Strauss, A. L., & Corbin, J. (1990). *Basics of qualitative research: Grounded theory procedures and techniques.* Newbury Park, CA: Sage.

von Wright, G. (1971). *Explanation and understanding.* London: Routledge & Kegan Paul.

This article was first published in the BMJ and is reproduced by permission of the BMJ.

Recognising meningococcal disease in primary care: qualitative study of how general practitioners process clinical and contextual information

Stephen Granier, Penny Owen, Roisin Pill, Lionel Jacobson

Department of General Practice and Primary Care, King's College School of Medicine and Dentistry, London SE5 9PJ

Stephen Granier, *research fellow* Llanedeyrn Health Centre, Cardiff CF3 7PN

Penny Owen, *general practitioner* Department of General Practice, University of Wales College of Medicine, Cardiff CF3 7PN

Roisin Pill, *professor* Lionel Jacobson, *research fellow*

Correspondence to: Dr Granier

BMJ 1998;316:276–9

Abstract

Objectives: To describe the presentation of meningococcal disease in primary care; to explore how general practitioners process clinical and contextual information in children with meningococcal disease; and to describe how this information affects management.
Design: Qualitative analysis of semistructured interviews.
Setting: General practices in South Glamorgan.
Subjects: 26 general practitioners who between January 1994 and December 1996 admitted 31 children (under 16 years of age) in whom meningococcal disease was diagnosed.
Main outcome measures: Categories of clinical rules and techniques used by general practitioners in processing each case.
Results: 22 children had rashes; in 16 of them the rashes were non–blanching. When present, a haemorrhagic rash was the most important factor in the doctor's decision to admit a child. 22 children had clinical features not normally expected in children with acute self limiting illnesses – for example, lethargy, poor eye contact, altered mental states, pallor with a high temperature, and an abnormal cry. Contextual information, such as knowledge of parents' consultation patterns and their normal degree of anxiety, played an important part in the management decisions in 15 cases. Use of penicillin was associated with the certainty of diagnosis and the presence and type of haemorrhagic rash.
Conclusion: The key clinical feature of meningococcal disease – a haemorrhagic rash – was present in only half of the study children. The general practitioners specifically hunted for the rash in some ill children, but doctors should not be deterred from diagnosing meningococcal disease and starting antibiotic treatment if the child is otherwise well, if the rash has an unusual or scanty distribution, or if the rash is non–haemorrhagic.

Introduction

Current knowledge on the presentation of meningococcal disease has been defined largely from the results of studies based in hospitals, where the disease is seen at a late stage.[1-8] General practitioners encounter meningococcal disease earlier, when signs and symptoms are often non–specific, making diagnosis difficult. Early treatment for meningococcal disease has been widely recommended and shown to improve outcome[7-11] in all but one study.[12] Prompt treatment requires early recognition, but in up to a quarter of cases the diagnosis is delayed by more than 48 hours after the onset of the illness.[1-13] A review of the published research on meningococcal disease found only one study on the recognition of meningococcal disease (predominantly meningitis of all types) using data from primary care.[14] Some studies reviewed referral letters,[6,7] but these are unlikely to carry full information because of the context in which the letters are written, at a time when rapid admission to hospital and initiation of antibiotic treatment are more urgent than the comprehensive recording of symptoms and signs. We explored how general practitioners made diagnostic and management decisions in children later found to have meningococcal disease. We used a qualitative approach to allow for in–depth exploration of the clinical and contextual features that general practitioners considered important and how this information was used in decision making.

Subjects and methods

We identified 83 cases of meningococcal disease in children and teenagers under 16 years old that occurred in two hospitals in South Glamorgan from January 1994 to December 1996 using hospital morbidity data. Cases without positive results on culture of blood or cerebrospinal fluid were included when a meningococcal disease had been diagnosed in hospital on the basis of the clinical presentation and course of the illness and when complete antibiotic treatment was given. We found hospital notes for 63 cases (76%), and we analysed general practitioner referral letters, admission clinical notes, and bacteriological data. Thirty one children were selected by purposive sampling so that the cases selected would represent the full range of presentations, management, and outcome. These children were referred by 26 general practitioners, who were interviewed using semi–structured audiotaped interviews.

All interviews were conducted by one of the authors (SG). The main part of the interview focused on the general practitioner's previous experiences of the disease, a description of the particular case, and the key features of the case that he or she had considered important in the management. These questions were refined during the pilot and study interviews. Interviews were transcribed word for word; in two cases, notes were taken: in one because the general practitioner preferred not to be recorded and in the other because the equipment failed. Copies of all transcripts were sent to the participants for clarification. Clinical information given by general practitioners was also verified by examination of referral letters and hospital notes. The data were assembled on a matrix using Word for Windows Version 6.0a to allow for comparison of categories for each interview. Patterns and differences were explored. The process was iterative, in that later interviews probed new emerging themes. Another of us (PO) helped validation by independently reading transcripts and listening to all interviews.

Results

All 26 general practitioners contacted agreed to participate. Their mean age was 42 years (range 29–55 years), and 10 were women. These data were similar to those for all general practitioners in South Glamorgan. Twenty four were principals in general practice, with a mean duration of 11 years' service. Fifteen were members of the Royal College of General Practitioners and 18 had undergone some postgraduate training in paediatrics. The mean interval between case and interview was 61 (SD 39) weeks. Nine general practitioners commented independently on how clearly the events remained in their minds, and the detailed descriptions of 10 others implied good recall. Four general practitioners had some difficulty in describing certain details, and three did not remember the cases very well, but they were able to refer to their clinical notes.

Our subsample of 31 children was similar to the total of 63 children admitted with meningococcal disease with regard to age and sex distribution, the number of times seen by a general practitioner before admission, the duration of illness before admission, the proportion with a rash on admission, and outcome (table).

Rashes
Non–blanching rash – Of the 31 children, 16 presented with haemorrhagic rashes. The presence of a non–blanching rash was the most important factor in

Comparison of general practice sample of 31 children with all 63 children admitted with meningococcal disease. Values are numbers (percentages) of patients

	General practice sample (n=31)	Hospital patients (n=63)
Age group:		
0–12 months	7 (23)	20 (32)
13–24 months	5 (16)	6 (10)
24 months–5 years	10 (32)	20 (32)
>5 years	9 (2)	17 (27)
Duration of illness (hours):		
0–24	23 (74)	44 (70)
25–48	2 (6)	11 (18)
>48	6 (19)	7 (11)
Missing data	0	1 (2)
No of contacts with GP during present illness (within 1 week):		
None	0	4 (6)
1	19 (61)	33 (52)
2	10 (32)	17 (27)
3–5	2 (7)	2 (3)
Missing data	0	7 (11)
Outcome:		
Full recovery	26 (84)	52 (83)
Neurological sequelae	2 (7)	2 (3)
Physical sequelae	0	2 (3)
Death	2 (7)	4 (6)
Still to be followed up	1 (3)	2 (3)
Missing data	0	1 (2)

deciding whether to admit these children. "He had an obvious purpuric rash starting on his legs and trunk, and it was clear what the diagnosis was . . . It's the rash you see in books" (general practitioner 1).

Other explanations – A purpuric rash influenced decisions to admit, but it also led to diagnostic difficulties. Henoch–Schönlein purpura was considered to be a more likely diagnosis in four children because the rash was present only on the legs, and one child without a fever was thought to have thrombocytopenic purpura.

Extent and distribution of the rash – In eight children the haemorrhagic rash was localised, most commonly on the legs or buttocks. In some cases it consisted of only one or a few spots. "I remember . . . examining him reasonably carefully, seeing a spot on his tummy . . . and prodding it with my finger . . . thinking it was a freckle. And I noticed it didn't blanch" (general practitioner 2).

Non–petechial rashes – Six children had blanching macular rashes. In four of these the doctors suspected the rash might be a marker of serious illness. Three were described as consisting of small red lesions, 1–2 mm in diameter, which blanched with pressure.

Abnormal illness
Twenty two children had clinical features not normally expected in children with acute self limiting febrile illnesses. Nine children were abnormally lethargic. Five were described as almost motionless and not wanting to be moved, while three children seemed to be vacant and

did not make eye contact or interact with their parents or the general practitioner. Five children had altered mental states: two were confused, two were behaving abnormally, and one was comatose. Three children had abnormal cries (either high or low pitched), one was crying inconsolably, five were pale, and three were cyanosed. "He was acting strangely, and Mum had said he had become aggressive, which was totally out of character for him" (general practitioner 3).

Puzzling findings

Unusual or puzzling findings were described in nine children. Two children were feverish but pale and with poor blood circulation. "Thinking about it, he was paler than he should have been for the temperature. That is the one thing that has stuck with me. He was boiling hot, but he wasn't red" (general practitioner 2). Two children were described as crying when handled, preferring not to be held. Four general practitioners reported being puzzled about children with joint pain, which led them to consider explanations for the illness other than acute self limiting causes. "He had a viral rash, macular rash, blanched on pressure, a bit sleepy, a bit irritable and complaining of pain in his knees and ankles, which was a bit odd" (general practitioner 4).

Misleading information

An apparent focal cause for a febrile illness was sometimes misleading – for example, infected tonsils in one child. In five cases an apparently well looking child was potentially misleading, in that most general practitioners expected children with the rash of meningococcal disease to be systemically unwell. "She was sat in that easy chair looking really, as I say, quite well. Not much different to how you look, frankly" (general practitioner 5).

Role of parents

Contextual information played an important part in the management decision in 15 cases. Most commonly, this entailed taking into account the context of the family and the perceived degree of parental anxiety, especially when the parents and their consulting patterns were well known to the general practitioner. This was of particular importance in eight of the 15 children who did not present with a non–blanching rash. "So she is a sensible mum – you know, comes along with appropriate problems – so it's nice to have that background. And she came with [her son] who had been irritable, off his feeds, and had vomited twice that morning and she burst into tears . . . So that was a major factor in my assessment of the child, I think" (general practitioner 6). "It's one I remember reasonably well and I suppose their family do stick out in your mind because I think she's got three young boys and it's fairly unique in that we would never have done a house call" (general practitioner 7). In two consultations parents played a part in prompting general practitioners to change their management plans. "Then Dad said he had noticed me prodding [a small petechial lesion] and said: 'What is that? I've not noticed that before.' And that was when I looked again" (general practitioner 2).

Management in primary care

Thirteen children were given intramuscular penicillin by their general practitioners before hospital admission. None received intravenous antibiotics. Certainty of meningococcal disease and the presence and type of haemorrhagic rash (no rash, localised rash, or widespread rash) were the most important predictors of the use of penicillin (x^2 for linear trend = 3.6 for certainty (df = 1, P < 0.01) and 4.5 for rash (df = 1, P < 0.05)). Penicillin was given in nine out of 13 cases in which general practitioners were completely certain of the diagnosis and in four out of nine cases in which they were moderately certain. All four children without haemorrhagic rashes who were given penicillin were considered to be very ill. Of these, two had macular rashes, which caused the general practitioners to suspect meningococcal disease, and two had evidence of meningeal irritation. "And so there I was with this extremely sick boy and I didn't, I really didn't have a clue what was wrong with him and the only thing that made me really seriously think about meningitis was the fact he'd had this ache in his neck the night before and that he'd become extremely ill quickly. . . . As meningitis was the only thing I could do anything about I gave him some penicillin" (general practitioner 7).

Neither paediatric training nor experience of meningococcal disease was associated with treatment, although penicillin was given in only one of the five cases in which general practitioners had no previous experience of meningococcal disease.

Discussion

The clinical information used in decision making by this sample of general practitioners was different from the clinical data described in studies of the presentation at the time of hospital admission.[1-6] Our qualitative interviews with general practitioners have shown that each child with meningococcal disease presented with a unique and often widely varying combination of clinical symptoms and contextual features. Analysis of these interviews has identified five common clinical rules and techniques that helped general practitioners process each unique dataset.

Clinical features

Firstly, we have confirmed the key clinical importance of a haemorrhagic rash in diagnosing meningococcal disease in children in primary care. A non–blanching rash was the most important independent factor leading to hospital admission and initiation of antibiotic treatment beforehand. This supports the findings of two previous studies.[7-10] Haemorrhagic rashes were found in just over half of the children, compared with around 70% of children under the age of 15 years in two hospital studies.[3-7] This difference may be accounted for by the rapid onset of rashes between assessment in primary care and assessment in hospital.

Secondly, whereas some children with rashes of meningococcal disease seemed to be well, a rash could have been missed if it was not specifically looked for in ill children. If a haemorrhagic rash is present general practitioners should not be deterred from diagnosing meningococcal disease when the child is otherwise well or when the distribution of the rash is unusual or scanty.[15] Our interviews show that meningococcal disease may present with a maculopapular rash.

Thirdly, general practitioners were aware of abnormal illness in children and detected features that did not apply to self limiting illnesses. Other children presented with features that were not dissimilar to those of self limiting illnesses, but they had unusual, odd, or puzzling findings which caused the general practitioner to consider a more serious cause for their illnesses.

Fourthly, awareness of parents' help–seeking behaviour played an important part in decision making. Responding to parents' impressions of their ill children was particularly helpful when the family was well known to the general practitioner.

Finally, general practitioners were prepared to discount certain potentially misleading information. For example, they were not deterred by a lack of parental concern or the child being otherwise well when undertaking an appropriately thorough assessment.

Implications for treatment

Our findings show that the recommendation that general practitioners start antibiotic treatment [16][17] is largely being followed when the diagnosis is certain. Failure to start treatment seems to be related to uncertainty about the diagnosis, partly because of the tendency to focus on extreme signs. It may be appropriate for general practitioners to use parenteral penicillin more readily in children requiring admission to hospital.

Poor response rates to postal questionnaires have been linked to a lack of perceived relevance of the research to general practitioners.[18] Our 100% response rate may indicate that general practitioners consider the diagnosis of meningococcal disease to be an important topic for research, as well as reflecting the acceptability of the method we used to collect data – namely, semistructured interviews with a fellow clinician. Our complex data would probably not have been obtained by a structured questionnaire. Many of the general practitioners welcomed the opportunity to discuss the events leading to admission. As this was a retrospective study, they could have reconstructed their experiences in keeping with management decisions and the outcome or portrayed their clinical decisions in a more favourable manner. However, some of them commented on how clearly the events remained in their minds.

> **KEY MESSAGES**
>
> • In primary care the main emphasis in managing meningococcal disease in children is early recognition and initiation of antibiotic treatment
>
> • In this study of 26 general practitioners admitting 31 children with meningococcal disease, a haemorrhagic rash was the most important single factor leading to admission but was present in only half of the children
>
> • When a haemorrhagic rash is present general practitioners should not be deterred from diagnosing meningococcal disease and starting antibiotic treatment if the child is otherwise well or if the rash is scanty or has an unusual distribution
>
> • The general practitioners noted abnormal illnesses with features different from those of acute self limiting illnesses, including unwillingness to interact or make eye contact, altered mental states, and pallor with a high temperature
>
> • Knowledge of parents and their help–seeking behaviour were important in making management decisions
>
> • General practitioners were prepared to discount potentially misleading information

We thank the general practitioners who gave their time to be interviewed for this study. We also thank Professor D P Davies and Drs R Verrier–Jones and P White for their constructive comments and advice, and Mrs H Sottero and Mrs G Jones for their help.

Contributors: SG initiated the primary study hypothesis, undertook the literature search, discussed core ideas, designed the study protocol, audited hospital records, conducted all qualitative interviews with the general practitioners, and participated in analysing data and writing the manuscript. PO had the original idea for the study, discussed core ideas, read the background literature, contributed to the study hypothesis and protocol, audited hospital records, and participated in analysing data and writing the manuscript. RP discussed core ideas, contributed to the design of the study protocol, and participated in analysing and interpreting data and in writing the manuscript. LJ discussed core ideas and contributed to the study hypothesis, design of the protocol, piloting, interpreting data, and writing and editing the manuscript. Christopher Butler and Nigel Stott discussed core ideas and contributed to the study protocol and editing of the manuscript. SG and PO are guarantors of the study.
Funding: None.
Conflict of interest: None.

References

1 Olcen P, Barr J, Kjellander J. Meningitis and bacteraemia due to Neiserria meningitidis: clinical and laboratory findings in 69 cases from Orebo county, 1965 to 1977. *Scand J Infect Dis* 1979;11:111–9.

2 Donald P, Burger P, van Zyl L. Meningococcal disease at Tygerburg Hospital. *S Afr Med J* 1980;60:271–5.

3 Palmer S, Corson J, Hall R, Payne S, Ludlow J, Deere B, et al. Meningococcal disease in Wales: clinical features, outcome and public health management. *J Infect* 1992;25:321–8.

[4] Voss L, Lennon D, Sinclair J. The clinical features of paediatric meningococcal disease, Auckland, 1985–87. *NZ Med J* 1989;102:243–5.

[5] Wong V, Hitchcock W, Mason W. Meningococcal infections in children: a review of 100 cases. *Pediatr Infect Dis J* 1989;8:224–7.

[6] Nielson B, Sorensen HT, Nielson JO. Children admitted for observation of suspected meningitis. *Scand J Primary Health Care* 1988;6:229–32.

[7] Woodward C, Jessop E, Wale M. Early management of meningococcal disease. *Commun Dis Rep CDR Rev* 1995;5(9):R135–7.

[8] Riordan F, Thomson A, Sills J, Hart CE. Who spots the spots? Diagnosis of early meningococcal disease in children. *BMJ* 1996;313:1255–6.

[9] Strang PR, Pugh EJ. Meningococcal infections: reducing the case fatality rate by giving penicillin before admission to hospital. *BMJ* 1992;305:141–3.

[10] Cartwright K, Reilly S, White D, Stuart J. Early treatment with parenteral penicillin in meningococcal disease. *BMJ* 1992;305:143–7.

[11] Cartwright K, Strang J, Gossain S, Begg N. Early treatment of meningococcal disease. *BMJ* 1992;305:774.

[12] Sorensen HT, Moller–Petersen K, Krarup HB, Pedersen H, Hansen H, Hamburger H. Early treatment of meningococcal disease. *BMJ* 1992;305:774.

[13] Kilpi T, Antilla M, Kallio M, Peltola H. Severity of childhood bacterial meningitis and duration of illness before diagnosis. *Lancet* 1991;338:406–9.

[14] Koorevaar R, Bruinzeels M, can der Wouden C, van der Velden K, van Suijlekom–Smit L. Patients with suspected meningitis: a study in general practice. *Eur J Gen Pract* 1995;1:21–4.

[15] Marzouk O, Thomson APJ, Sills JA, Hart CA, Harris F. Features and outcome in meningococcal disease presenting with maculopapular rash. *Arch Dis Child* 1991;66:486–7.

[16] Department of Health and Social Security. *Meningococcal infection: meningitis and septicaemia*. London: HMSO, 1988. (CMO(88)2.)

[17] Cartwright K, Strang J, Reilly S, White D. Mortality in meningococcal disease. *BMJ* 1992;304:116.

[18] McAvoy B, Kaner E. General practice postal surveys: a questionnaire too far. *BMJ* 1989;313:732–3.

(Accepted 28 October 1997)

ARTICLE 4

HEALTH BELIEFS AND FOLK MODELS OF DIABETES IN BRITISH BANGLADESHIS: A QUALITATIVE STUDY

Trisha Greenhalgh, Cecil Helman, A Mu'min Chowdhury

Qualitative Research Unit, Joint Department of Primary Care and Population Sciences, University College London Medical School/ Royal Free Hospital School of Medicine, Whittington Hospital, London N19 5NF

Trisha Greenhalgh, *senior lecturer*
Cecil Helman, *senior lecturer*
A Mu'min Chowdhury, *research fellow*
Correspondence to: Dr Greenhalgh p.greenhalgh@ucl.ac.uk
BMJ 1998;316:978–83

ARTICLE 5

Abstract

Objective: To explore the experience of diabetes in British Bangladeshis, since successful management of diabetes requires attention not just to observable behaviour but to the underlying attitudes and belief systems which drive that behaviour.

Design: Qualitative study of subjects' experience of diabetes using narratives, semi–structured interviews, focus groups, and pile sorting exercises. A new qualitative method, the structured vignette, was developed for validating researchers' understanding of primary level culture.

Subjects: 40 British Bangladeshi patients with diabetes, and 10 non–Bangladeshi controls, recruited from primary care.

Result: Several constructs were detected in relation to body image, cause and nature of diabetes, food classification, and knowledge of complications. In some areas, the similarities between Bangladeshi and non–Bangladeshi subjects were as striking as their differences. There was little evidence of a fatalistic or deterministic attitude to prognosis, and most informants seemed highly motivated to alter their diet and comply with treatment. Structural and material barriers to behaviour change were at least as important as "cultural" ones.

Conclusion: Bangladeshi culture is neither seamless nor static, but some widely held beliefs and behaviours have been identified. Some of these have a potentially beneficial effect on health and should be used as the starting point for culturally sensitive diabetes education.

Introduction

Successful management of diabetes requires that we understand the lifestyle, beliefs, attitudes, and family and social networks of the patients being treated.[1] Qualitative methods are particularly useful when the subject of research is relatively unexplored and the research question is loosely defined or open ended.[2] With two recently published exceptions[3 4] and a small British study based entirely on individual interviews,[5] such methods have rarely been used in the study of diabetes.

Anthropological analysis accepts that there are three levels of cultural behaviour: what people say they do (for example, during an interview), what they are actually observed to do, and the underlying belief system which drives that behaviour (Hall's "primary level culture"[6]). In addition, consideration must be given to the wider context in which the behaviour takes place. In particular, the British Bangladeshi informants in this study must be viewed as members of an atomistic rural society living as recent immigrants in a socio-economically deprived urban environment (see box).

Bangladeshi population of East London

The frontiers of present day Bangladesh were drawn after the second world war, when British India was partitioned. The Muslim majority of Bengal, along with Sylhet district in the far north east, came to form East Pakistan. In 1971 Bengal seceded from Pakistan and became the separate state of Bangladesh. The country is flat, with a monsoon climate, prone to flooding, and served mainly by inland waterways. The economy is pre–industrial, and most people live in scattered homesteads with an atomistic social organisation (that is, the family is the dominant unit with no effective social organisation or hierarchy beyond the family). The staple crop is rice, and the diet is largely fish, rice, and vegetables. Although about 95% of the population is Muslim, the society contains vestiges of its Buddhist and Hindu cultural roots. In the 1960s and '70s, large numbers of economic migrants came to Britain, particularly from certain villages in rural Sylhet. Men tended to emigrate several years before their wives followed. Data from the 1991 census suggest that British Bangladeshis account for about 0.3% of the population of England and Wales,[7] and about a quarter of the population of Tower Hamlets (East London and City Health Authority; unpublished estimates for 1997 based on projections from 1991 census data).

Subjects and methods

Subjects

After gaining approval from local research ethics committees, we recruited patients from three general practices in east London known to have a high proportion of Bangladeshi patients. Using computerised diabetes registers where available, and otherwise by manual search of case notes, we identified patients with diabetes and approached them to request a tape recorded interview. Recruitment was usually by letter followed up by telephone call, but in one practice we recruited opportunistically through practice receptionists when patients came to book appointments or collect prescriptions. In all, 40 of the 44 Bangladeshi subjects we approached agreed to be interviewed.

We interviewed these 40 Bangladeshis and a control group of eight white British and two Afro–Caribbean subjects who lived in east London and had similar socioeconomic background. We used purposive sampling methods (that is, we intentionally sought to interview subjects with certain characteristics) to ensure a range of demographic variables and experiences (see table 1).

Methods

The research methods used are summarised in the box. We allowed the subjects to tell their story in their own words and in no particular order, but we used a checklist of semistructured prompting questions to make sure that the domains listed in the box were covered at some stage by all subjects.

Translation

Interviews with Bangladeshi subjects were conducted in Sylheti, a dialect of Bengali spoken as a first language by all our Bangladeshi subjects. Since Sylheti has no written form, the interviews were simultaneously translated and transcribed by an independent translator and were all checked by AMC (a Sylheti anthropologist), who listened to the original recording while reading the draft translation.

Analysis

Transcripts were analysed with nudist software. The entire text of the interview was entered onto a computer database and text blocks were coded into 11 broad categories of statement such as body image, information sources, professional roles, and so on.

The objective of the analysis was to identify constructs – that is, provisional inferences about primary level culture drawn from statements and observations.[9] Using the powerful cross referencing facility of the software, we considered together all statements relevant to each construct and modified the construct accordingly.

Validation

An important technique for demonstrating the validity of qualitative findings is triangulation – comparing data obtained by one method with similar data obtained by another method.[10] After developing the constructs, we

Table 1 Characteristics of subjects interviewed in qualitative study

	Bangladeshi (n=40)	Non–Bangladeshi (n=10)
Age (years)		
21–40	6	0
41–60	23	5
61–80	11	5
Education		
None	13	0
<3 years school	15	0
>3 years school	10	10
Higher	2	0
Employment		
Employed	1	2
Unemployed	16	3
Housewife	15	1
Pensioner	8	4
Housing		
Owner occupied	2	1
Council rented	38	9
Language		
Sylheti only	24	0
Sylheti plus standard Bengali	8	0
Sylheti plus standard Bengali plus English	8	0
English only	0	10
Type of diabetes (method of control)		
Diet alone	6	1
Diet plus tablets	32	6
Diet plus insulin	2	3
Generation of immigrant		
Indigenous	0	9
First	39	1
Second	1	0
Extended family in United Kingdom		
Yes	33	8
No	7	2
Known diabetes complications		
Yes	21	4
No	19	5
Missing data	0	1
Type of care		
General practitioner only	15	3
Shared (general practitioner plus hospital)	25	7
Hospital only	0	0

presented them to a smaller sample of the subjects to determine whether our interpretation of the initial interviews had been correct. For this, we used two methods, the first being a further set of sex specific focus groups in which we presented our initial constructs and recorded the group's responses on videotape. In the second, we developed the new qualitative technique of structured vignette.

Structured vignette – We presented our constructs in the form of a story recorded on tape about Mr (or Mrs) Ali, a person with diabetes. The story was first played in full and then played back slowly, sentence by sentence. After each sentence, the tape was stopped and the subject asked: "Do you agree that this person would have [acted in this way/thought this/etc]?" (A sample paragraph of the vignette is reproduced in the appendix.) The vignette

Qualitative methods used in study

Audiotaped narrative in which subject "tells the story" of his or her diabetes (all subjects)

Semistructured interview in which defined domains are covered (all subjects), including

Personal medical history
Psychological reaction to diagnosis of diabetes
Knowledge about causes, complications and treatment
     objectives in diabetes
Body image and beliefs about physiological and
     pathological processes
Attitude to dietary restriction
Attitude to physical exercise
Perceived social constraints resulting from diabetes
Satisfaction with current diabetes service
Experience of, and attitude to, health professionals

Focus group discussion of 6–9 participants grouped by sex, in which similar topics are covered and areas of controversy and dissent within the group specifically explored (total of 24 subjects)

Construction of genogram ("family tree") (all subjects)

Pile sorting exercises (all subjects), comprising

Disease ranking—Diabetes is ranked against 10 other
     medical conditions (heart attack, gastric ulcer, flu,
     asthma, gall stones, back pain, tuberculosis, cancer,
     stroke, and malaria)
Foods—Raw foodstuffs are grouped into "permitted" and
     "not permitted" and the classification then discussed
Meal menus—Above exercise is repeated with complete
     meals
"Preferred" and "healthy" body size—A selection of eight
     photographs of Bangladeshis (all of similar age and
     same sex as informant but of varying body mass index)
     is sorted into "most [aesthetically] preferred" through
     to "least preferred" and again into "most healthy"
     through to "least healthy"

Structured vignette method (see text for details) (18 subjects)

Feedback of preliminary constructs to focus groups, in which responses were videotaped (eight subjects)

Study of patients' general practice case notes (the "Lloyd George" record), which also contain correspondence about hospital admissions and outpatient visits (all subjects)

included some deliberately incorrect statements to check that subjects were not simply agreeing with all the statements. This method was developed to avoid the problems, which have been well documented in non–European cultures,[11] of asking informants to respond to closed questions about their own beliefs or behaviour, which would require them to challenge directly statements made by the interviewer. We performed the structured vignette study on a sample of 18 subjects, and repeated it on 10 of these same subjects after an interval of two months. The internal reliability of the technique was high (overall, 89% of questions received identical answers on repeat interview).

Results

Sources of explanatory models

The desire of the informants to understand and explain the onset and experience of illness was often strong. However, it tended not to lead to a systematic search for professional or scientific explanations but rather to a reflection on personal experience and the experiences of friends and relatives. Lay sources of information were frequently cited as a major influence on behaviour. In the structured vignette study, 17 of the 18 informants agreed that the best way to find out about diabetes was to ask friends and relatives.

While strong religious (Muslim) views were held by all the Bangladeshi informants and explanations often given in terms of "God's will," such views were usually held in parallel with acceptance of individual responsibility and potential for change. Indeed, both stoicism and adherence to particular dietary choices were perceived as the duty of the ill person.

Constructs

Body concepts

Youth and health were usually viewed as virtually synonymous, and physical degeneration and weakness as an inevitable consequence of aging – "Once you are 40 eyes tend to give trouble. I am almost 55. So I am expected to have bad eyesight" (Bangladeshi man).

In contrast, Crawford's study of white women in the United States indicated that "health" for them was not merely the absence of illness but had to be earned by taking positive action in terms of diet and exercise in leisure time. [12]

Both men and women chose photographs of large individuals when asked to "pick out the healthiest person." Large body size was generally viewed as an indicator of "more health" and thinness with "less health," but many also perceived that "too much health" (that is, too large a body size) was undesirable, especially if the body is weakened by diabetes. Airhihenbuwa has discussed the phenomenon of immigrants holding simultaneously both "traditional" constructs (deeply rooted values and perceptions drawn from the culture of origin) and "recent" ones (drawn from the host culture and less likely to be enduring in the long term).[13]

Origin and nature of diabetes

Illness was generally attributed to events or agents ouside the body rather than to primary failure of an organ within it. This model may reflect the predominance of acute infectious illness in the recent cultural history of this group. All informants believed that the primary cause of diabetes, and that of poor diabetic control, was too much sugar and, to a lesser extent, other features of a Western diet, both of which feature strongly in folk models of other cultural groups.[2 4 14 15]

Other aetiological factors mentioned by the Bangladeshi informants included heredity (the notion of an agent transmitted through "shared blood" rather than an inherited predisposition) and germs. Many inform–ants mentioned physical or psychological stress, either as a perceived cause of diabetes or simply when reporting the experience of daily life – especially in relation to economic difficulties, poor housing, and fear of crime.

Impact of diabetes

The diagnosis of diabetes was generally seen as devastating, and the expression "I was spoiled" was used by several informants. Virtually all felt that diabetes was a chronic, incurable condition and a potential threat to life. They feared acute complications (collapse and "dropping dead"), and a minority volunteered specific long term sequelae in the heart, eyes, and kidneys. Control of diabetes (and therefore reduction in disability and prolongation of life) was felt to lie in restoring the body's internal balance via taking particular foods and fighting the "germ" with medicine.

Many informants expressed difficulty obtaining food that was both acceptable and palatable. Other practical difficulties included confusion over sickness benefits; language barriers when speaking to professionals, especially the use of children as interpreters; and the inability to understand leaflets, either because of the concepts presented or because the leaflets were printed in standard Bengali (some informants said they were better able to understand the English alphabet, such as in road signs or notices, than standard Bengali).

Diet and nutrition

In the pile sorting exercise, foods were not grouped according to Western notions of nutritional content but in terms of their perceived strength (nourishing power) and digestibility. "Strong" foods, perceived as energy giving, included white sugar, lamb, beef, ghee (derived from butter), solid fat, and spices. Such foods were considered health giving and powerful for the healthy body and suitable for festive occasions, but liable to produce worsening of illness in the old or debilitated. "Weak" foods, preferred in the everyday menu and for the old or infirm, included boiled (pre–fluffed) rice and cereals.

Raw foods, and those that had been baked or grilled, were considered indigestible, as were any vegetables that grew under the ground. Foods of low digestibility were considered unsuitable for elderly, debilitated, or young people. Thus, the recommendation for diabetic patients to bake or grill foods rather than fry them may not accord with cultural perceptions of digestibility.

The structured vignette study showed almost universal agreement that strong foods, solid fat, and ghee should be avoided in diabetes. All 18 agreed that Mr Ali should not eat spicy foods because of his diabetes and that a person with diabetes should eat a different diet from the rest of the family.

Some informants indicated that body components may be linked to certain foods because of physical similarity. For example, sugar, butter, ghee, body fat, bone marrow, semen, and white vaginal discharge were perceived by some to be the same fundamental entity, because their colour is the same and they all solidify when cool and liquefy when heated. Eight of 18 informants in the structured vignette study thought that molasses (a dark form of raw sugar, liquid at room temperature) was an acceptable substitute for sugar in the diet.

"Sugar is the white substance that is stored in the bone marrow, is it not? From this semen is produced. Since I have diabetes, I have come to think that [it is] because of using the semen more. When the 'calcium' inside the bone is exhausted at that time our diabetes starts" (Bangladeshi man in focus group). This statement brought general agreement in the focus group. These findings are consistent with Lambert's work on the traditional South Asian "humoral" concepts of health, which centre on the ecological flow of substances and qualities between the environment, food, and the human body.[16]

Many informants believed that the same amount of rice could be taken as frequent small meals since it was imbalance, rather than total quantity, that mattered. In the structured vignette study, 16 of 18 informants agreed that Mr Ali's doctor had underestimated the amount of rice he needed when advising him to reduce his food intake, and all 18 agreed he should take biscuits or other snacks between meals to sustain his strength. Only five thought that such snacks could cause any harm.

In Bangladeshi society, feasts, festivals, and social occasions are common, culturally important, and centre on eating sweet and rich food. A calculated compromise between dietary compliance and social duty was usually made.

Smoking

Of our Bangladeshi informants, nine of the 23 men and none of the 17 women smoked; only a few took paan (chewing tobacco) regularly, and those who did acknowledged that it was harmful and expressed a desire to quit. In the structured vignette study, only four of 18 informants disagreed that tobacco was harmful.

Concepts of balance

Many cultures equate balance with health and imbalance with illness.[17] There was a strong and almost universal belief among the Bangladeshi informants that both the onset and the control of diabetes depended on the balance of food entering the body and on balanced emission of body fluids such as sweat, semen, urine, menstrual blood, etc. Excess emission was perceived to deplete the internal stock, low quantity of emissions to indicate inner build up and putrefaction, and thin quality a weakening of the internal stock. Weakness (as in diabetes) was perceived to occur as a result of such depletion or weakening.

Absence of sweating (due to the cold British climate and lack of physical labour) on immigration to Britain was commonly cited as a cause of diabetes and a reason why the condition improved or disappeared on return to hot countries. In the structured vignette study, 14 of 18 informants agreed that if Mr Ali returned to Bangladesh his diabetes might be cured.

Exercise
Exercise in the context of health and fitness seemed to have little cultural meaning for the Bangladeshi informants, even though they often recalled specific advice on this topic from their doctor. Exercise was viewed as potentially exacerbating illness or physical weakness. The association between sweating (see above) and exercise in leisure time was not made by any informant, but ritual Muslim prayers (namaz) were often cited as a worthy and health giving form of exercise.

The Sylheti language has no expression for physical activity that has the same connotations of vitality, improvement in body condition, social desirability, and inherent "moral" value as the word "exercise." Sports and games are not generally pursued by adults in Bangladesh[18] or by Bangladeshis in Britain.[19] The closest translation for the word "exercise" is "beyam," a word of obscure etymology. Interestingly, the prefix "bey" in Sylheti often has negative connotations – for example, "beyaram" (meaning illness, literally "no comfort") or "beytamiz" (poor etiquette, literally "no manners") – and we were struck by the lack of positive connotations accorded to the concept by our Bangladeshi informants compared with the white British and Afro–Caribbeans.

Some informants gave physical or material constraints to taking exercise. In particular, many of the women rarely left their house, apparently through fear of physical attack. Some informants lived in high rise flats with no working lift, and some commented on the absence of parks, dirty pavements, and street crime.

Professional roles
The doctor was viewed as a busy, authoritative and knowledgeable person who rarely makes mistakes and has full understanding of the conditions he or she treats. Several informants felt that the doctor's instructions should always be obeyed, and 12 of 18 in the structured vignette study agreed that "Mr Ali's doctor [general practitioner] knows everything about diabetes." Twelve also agreed that it would be impertinent for Mr Ali to ask the doctor any questions. In contrast, both white British and Afro–Caribbean informants were openly assertive and critical of health professionals. Nurses were sometimes viewed in a traditional caring and technical role but were sometimes recognised as providers of information and advice.

Diabetic monitoring
Informants generally tested their urine regularly, and all who did so seemed to understand the importance of a change in the colour of the test strip. Most informants seemed to believe that, in the absence of symptoms, diabetes was well controlled. The need for regular surveillance when asymptomatic was rarely acknowledged, and only one of 18 informants in the structured vignette study thought that Mr Ali should ever visit the doctor if he did not feel ill. Preventive care was not well understood – "He [the doctor] explained to me and said before complications start, start wearing glasses. This is because your eyes are all right. The diabetes may affect either your eyes or your feet. So if you take the glasses, your eyes may be spared" (Bangladeshi man).

Discussion
Strengths and limitations of the study
This study addressed an important and previously underexplored subject in health research.[20] We used a wide range of qualitative techniques on a sample that is likely to have included the least acculturated members of British Bangladeshi society, since we recruited from practices with Bangladeshi general practitioners, nurses, or advocates, we required neither literacy (in any language) nor spoken English or Bengali for participation in the study (indeed, 24 of the 40 informants spoke only the Sylheti dialect), and the response rate for the individual interviews was high (91%). Furthermore, our main field worker was an experienced anthropologist who has worked with this community for 25 years and speaks Sylheti as his first language.

The sample does, however, have limitations. In recruiting subjects from general practices, we failed to access those who do not seek or receive Western medicine in any form. We recruited only one second generation Bangladeshi, probably for demographic reasons. We did not assess any measure of diabetic control in our informants (such as glycated haemoglobin, which was inconsistently recorded in case notes) so we were unable to relate individual perceptions or experiences to level of control.

Implications for policy and practice
Although the differences in body image and illness maps shown here are of considerable anthropological interest, we believe that our findings support the notion that the similarities in health beliefs and health related behaviours (for example, failed attempts to lose weight or give up smoking) between minority groups and the host culture are often understated and may be of more practical importance than their differences.[21]

ARTICLE 5

A recurring theme in this research was that of structural and material barriers to improving health. Poor housing, unsafe streets, and financial hardship were at least as important in preventing certain outcomes (such as taking regular exercise) as religious restrictions or ethnic customs, a finding noted by other researchers in this area.[21][22] It is not within the remit of this paper to expand on the profound socioeconomic disadvantage of many British Bangladeshis, nor on the literature linking poverty with health inequalities in general,[23] but the importance of this factor as a barrier to health gain should not be ignored.

Health education that concords with people's "lay epidemiology" and folk models is more likely to lead to changes in behaviour than that which seems to contradict such models. Airhihenbuwa and colleagues, in the context of AIDS prevention, have exposed the fallacy of the assumption that health education is merely a matter of determining "deficiencies" in knowledge and meeting those deficiencies with educational material such as leaflets, teaching seminars, or mass media programmes. Instead, educators must centralise the cultural experiences of those who have hitherto been marginalised.[13][24] Given that the Bangladeshis in this study indicated a high regard for oral explanations from informal sources (friends, relatives, and other patients with diabetes), we think that the potential for learning via oral sources within Bangladeshi culture is high.

Hence, rather than designing an education programme to be delivered externally to rectify "deficiencies" in knowledge or "incorrect" behaviour,[25] we suggest that health promotion programmes attempt to build on those beliefs, attitudes, and behaviours already existing in Bangladeshi culture that promote good diabetes control, prevent complications, and improve quality of life, and address practical barriers to positive health behaviours such as nonavailability of particular foodstuffs. The box lists examples of constructs which, though not universally held, are sufficiently prevalent in Bangladeshi culture to form the starting point for successful culturally sensitive health education and promotion.

Table 2 draws on a framework developed by Danial and Green to identify perceptual, structural, and reinforcing factors that influence specific behavioural

Constructs which might be used as starting points for culturally sensitive diabetes education in British Bangladeshis

• Diabetes is caused by sweet things, a Western diet, and stress
• Diabetes is chronic and incurable, but its effects can be lessened by changes in lifestyle
• Dietary modification is essential for diabetes control, and effort must be made to prepare special food for the family member with diabetes
• A person with diabetes should aim to lose weight if overweight
• Physical labour which produces sweat is beneficial to health
• Sugar, fatty food, and solid fat (including ghee derived from butter) are harmful
• Complications may occur if diabetes is poorly controlled
• Poor diabetic control can be detected by change in the colour of the urine testing strip

outcomes in health promotion.[26] We have used the recommendation for regular, low intensity, physical exercise as an example of a desired behavioural priority for people with diabetes. As table 2 shows, many of the constructs identified in our fieldwork have direct implications for educators working on an individual or public health level. In addition, however, this framework highlights both the broader social and political context within which behaviour change in minority ethnic groups must be placed, and the danger of assuming that "non-compliance" with such advice about lifestyle is always attributable to "cultural factors."

Contributors: TG conceptualised and supervised the study, helped with fieldwork, analysed and interpreted the data, and wrote the paper. AMC performed the fieldwork and data entry and analysed and interpreted the data. CH provided general advice and contributed to analysis and interpretation of the data. TG is guarantor for the paper. Funding: The salaries of TG and AMC for this study were covered by a Health Services Research Grant from the Wellcome Trust. Conflict of interest: None.

Appendix: Sample section from structured vignette

Statement	Agree	Disagree	Not sure	Comment
Mr Ali thought that living in Britain had caused his diabetes				
He thought that if he went back to Bangladesh the diabetes might be cured				
He thought that the lack of sweating in Britain was unhealthy and that it predisposed people to get diabetes				
He also thought that diabetes was caused by something that got into his body, like a germ or some other bad thing from outside				

Table 2 Examples of Bangladeshi patients' perceptions, structural and material barriers, and reinforcing factors affecting acceptance of a behavioural priority in diabetes education—"People with diabetes should take regular sustained low–intensity physical exercise"

Perceptions	Implications for health education and health policy
Loss of body sweat, such as occurs during physical labour, is good for health	Recommendations for physical exercise should focus on the potential for producing sweat in ways other than physical labour
Prayers (namaz) are a form of physical exercise	Educators should be aware of the perceived association of prayer with exercise
Sport and organised physical exercise have no cultural meaning and are inappropriate for women and older men. Sports clothing and footwear are "not appropriate for our community"	Non–sporting activities that do not require special clothing or footwear may be more acceptable than pressure to become involved in sport
Walking is an acceptable form of exercise, but fast walking is inappropriate, especially for women and those of high social status	Promotion of walking and other indigenous activities may allow activity level to be increased in a culturally acceptable way, at least for males
Women should generally remain within the home, dress modestly, and remain demure. Young children should remain with their mother or grandmother at all times	Activities that can be done discretely and in private (such as home exercise videos) may be more acceptable to women
Structural and material factors	
Walking in the street is considered unsafe, particularly for women and elderly people, because of fear of crime and harassment	Effective local and national policies on crime and racial harassment, and community policing in particular, are required on health as well as social grounds
Opportunities for exercise in daily living often go unrecognised	Health promotion campaigns should encourage walking to school and shops rather than using motor transport
Reinforcing factors	
Advice from educators and health professionals is held in high regard	Even though physical exercise is not part of the culture, it should be encouraged in individual doctor–patient encounters
Approval or disapproval by family seems to strongly influence lifestyle choices	Involvement of key family members in education for exercise is likely to improve its success

References

1 Bradley C, Gamsu DS, for the Psychological Well–being Working Group of the WHO/IDF St Vincent Declaration Action Programme for Diabetes. Measures of psychological well–being and treatment satisfaction developed from the responses of people with tablet–treated diabetes. *Diabet Med* 1994;7:510–6.

2 Helman CG. Research in primary care—the qualitative approach. In: Norton PG, Stewart M, Tudiver F, Bass MJ, Dunn E, eds. *Primary care research: traditional and innovative approaches.* London: Sage Publications, 1991:105–24.

3 Gittelsohn J, Harris SB, Burris KL, Kakegamic L, Landman L, Sharma A, et al. Use of ethnographic methods for applied research on diabetes among the Ojibway–Cree in Northern Ontario. *Health Educ Q* 1996;23:365–82.

4 Grams G, Herbert C, Heffernan C, Calam B, Wilson MA, Grzybowski S, et al. Haida perspectives on living with non–insulin–dependent diabetes. *Can Med Assoc J* 1996;155:1563–8.

5 Kelleher D, Islam S. "How should I live?" Bangladeshi people and non–insulin dependent diabetes. In: Kelleher D, Hillier S, eds. *Researching cultural differences in health.* London: Routeledge, 1996:220–37.

6 Hall ET. *Beyond culture.* New York: Anchor Books, 1977.

7 Balarajan R, Soni Raleigh V. The ethnic populations of England and Wales: the 1991 census. *Health Trends* 1992;24:113–6.

8 Kitzinger J. The methodology of focus groups: the importance of interaction between research participants. *Sociol Health Illness* 1994;16:104–21.

9 Hayes BE. How to measure empowerment. *Qual Progress* 1994;Feb:41–6.

10 Denzin NK, Lincoln YS, eds. *Handbook of qualitative research.* London: Sage Publications, 1994.

[11] Helman C. *Culture, health and illness.* 3rd ed. Oxford: Butterworth–Heinemann, 1994.

[12] Crawford R. A cultural account of "health": control, release and the social body. In: McKinley JB, ed. *Issues in the political economy of health care.* London: Tavistock, 1984:60–103.

[13] Airhihenbuwa CO. Developing culturally appropriate health programs. In: *Health and culture: beyond the Western paradigm.* London: Sage Publications, 1995:25–43.

[14] Pierce MB. Non–insulin dependent diabetes and its complications – beliefs, perceptions and prospects for risk reduction [thesis]. London: University of London, 1997.

[15] Garro L. Individual or societal responsibility? Explanations of diabetes in an Anishaabe (Ojibway) community. *Soc Sci Med* 1995;40:37–46.

[16] Lambert H. The cultural logic of Indian medicine: prognosis and etiology in Rajastani popular therapeutics. *Soc Sci Med* 1992;34:1069–76.

[17] Helman C. Balance and imbalance. In: *Culture, health and illness.* 3rd ed. Oxford: Butterworth–Heinemann, 1994:21–4.

[18] Chowdhury AM. Household kin and community in a Bangladesh village [thesis]. Exeter: University of Exeter, 1986.

[19] Health Education Authority. *Health and lifestyles survey: black and minority ethnic groups in England.* London, HEA, 1994.

[20] Greenhalgh PM. Diabetes in British south Asians—nature, nurture and culture. *Diabet Med* 1997;11:10–4.

[21] Lambert H, Rose H. Disembodied knowledge? Making sense of medical science. In: Irwin A, Wynne B, eds. *Misunderstanding science: Making sense of science and technology within everyday life.* Cambridge: Cambridge University Press, 1996:65–83.

[22] Anderson JM, Wiggins S, Rajwani R, Holbrook A, Blue C, Ng M. Living with a chronic illness: Chinese–Canadian and Euro–Canadian women with diabetes—exploring factors that influence management. *Soc Sci Med* 1995;41:181–95.

[23] Calman KC. Equity, poverty, and health for all. *BMJ* 1997;314:1187–91.

[24] Airhihenbuwa CO, Di Clemente RJ, Wingwood GM, Lowe A. HIV/AIDS education and prevention among African–Americans: a focus on culture. *AIDS Educ Prev* 1992;4:267–76.

[25] Becker MH. The tyranny of health promotion. *Public Health Rev* 1986;14:15–25.

[26] Danial M, Green LW. Application of the precede–proceed model in prevention and control of diabetes: a case illustration from an aboriginal community. *Diabet Spectrum* 1995;8:80–123.

(Accepted 2 February 1998)

This article was first published in the BMJ and is reproduced by permission of the BMJ.

WHAT WORRIES PARENTS WHEN THEIR PRESCHOOL CHILDREN ARE ACUTELY ILL AND WHY: A QUALITATIVE STUDY
Joe Kai

Department of Primary Health Care, Medical School, University of Newcastle upon Tyne, Newcastle upon Tyne NE2 4HH

Joe Kai, *lecturer in primary health care*

BMJ 1996;313:983-6

ABSTRACT

Objective – To identify and explore parents' concerns when young children become acutely ill.
Design – Qualitative study making use of semi-structured one to one and group interviews with parents of preschool children.
Setting – Disadvantaged inner city community.
Subjects – 95 parents of preschool children.
Results – Fever, cough, and the possibility of meningitis were parents' primary concerns when their children became acutely ill. Parents' concerns reflected lay beliefs, their interpretation of medical knowledge, and their fears that their child might die or be permanently harmed. Parents worried about failing to recognise a serious problem. Concerns were expressed within the context of keenly felt pressure, emphasising parents' responsibility to protect their child from harm. They were grounded in two linked factors: parents' sense of personal control when faced with illness in their child and the perceived threat posed by an illness.
Conclusions – Better understanding of parents' concerns may promote effective communication between health professionals and parents. Modification of parents' personal control and perceived threat using appropriate information and education that acknowledge and address their concerns may be a means of empowering parents.

INTRODUCTION

Children under 5 years old form the largest proportion of reactive workload in primary care,[1] with those from disadvantaged backgrounds having the highest contact rates[1-3] and morbidity.[4] Parents inevitably worry about their children when they are ill. Gaining an understanding of what parents worry about is important if parents' anxieties are to be addressed effectively and if relevant information and education is to be offered. Previous work has described the beliefs and behaviours of mothers with young children but has paid less attention to what provokes concern for parents when their children are acutely ill.[5-8] In this study and the accompanying paper[9] I sought to identify what worries parents when their children become acutely ill and to understand what motivates their concerns.

SUBJECTS AND METHODS

I conducted pilot interviews initially with parents who were patients registered on the shared list of my general practice. I then recruited parents who were not my patients and had at least one child under 5 years old from a range of community settings in a disadvantaged area: a community centre, a hostel for single mothers, another inner city general practice, and three parent and toddler groups.

One to one interviews – Parents attending the community centre and parents living in the hostel were invited to participate in the research by a community worker. A random one in four sample of mothers registered with the general practice was sent a postal invitation. Purposeful sampling[10 11] was then used to select willing parents for interview. Initially, parents from each of the three settings who might have had typical experiences (no specific characteristics) were interviewed. As the research progressed, I selected parents registered with the general practice who were thought to have particular experiences of caring for ill children and those who were thought to have atypical experiences after discussion with the practice. Such parents were actively sought to ensure that data and its interpretation were not distorted to one perspective and that all cases could be accommodated within the developing analysis. Sampling was intended to provide a range of experiences and perceptions so that the breadth of findings and concepts emerging might be understood. Table 1 describes those features of the resulting sample. The interviews were open ended, semi-structured, and conducted in parents' homes.

Focus group interviews – All parents attending three parent and toddler groups were invited by their group organisers to form a volunteer sample to participate in focus group interviews.[12] These were held where they usually met with the help of crèche facilities. Both one to one and group interviews were used to enhance the sufficiency and quality of data and facilitate comparison and confirmation of emerging concepts across different settings.

Data analysis – The interviews explored broad areas identified in the pilot but concentrated on encouraging parents to discuss freely what was important to them when coping with ill young children and how and why they thought as they did. All interviews were audiotaped

Table 1
Purposeful sample of parents in one to one interviews

Key characteristic of family interviewed	No of mothers (n=28)
Single mother in temporary hostel accommodation	4*
Child with chronic problems (asthma, epilepsy)	4
Child admitted with acute illness in previous 12 months	3
Child with special needs (Down's syndrome, tuberous sclerosis)	2
Frequent user of general practitioner's out of hours service	5†
Mother with health professional background	3‡
Others with preschool child or children	7

*Two aged 16, one aged 18, one aged 25.
†Two or more out of hours visits by general practitioner to ill children under 5 years old in past 12 months.
‡One auxiliary nurse, one registered general nurse, one health service manager (sample included four fathers).

and transcribed verbatim. Data collection and analysis were guided by grounded theory methodology.[13] Transcriptions were analysed to identify concepts and categories embedded within them. Concepts and their relations were confirmed, modified, or discarded from ongoing analysis by re-examination of earlier data and during subsequent data collection and analysis. Interviewing continued until no new concepts were being generated. This suggested that the findings and conceptual scheme developed were a valid picture of parents' concerns and perceptions.

Study sample – Ninety five parents were interviewed in total. Of parents invited to participate in the one to one interviews, 16 of the 22 mothers at the community centre, all four parents at the hostel, and 29 of the 47 mothers registered with the general practice agreed. Ultimately, 32 parents were selected and interviewed at home (24 mothers alone and four mothers with their male partners). A further 63 mothers (of 82 attending the parent and toddler groups) participated in 10 focus groups (range 5-8 mothers). All the interviews lasted between one and two hours and were conducted over a period of 14 months. Most parents were from socioeconomically disadvantaged backgrounds. All were white and English speaking. The mean age of mothers was 26 years (range 16-41 years). The characteristics of participants are summarised in tables 1 and 2.

Respondent validation – To establish that the dataset was complete and parents' experiences were fully described, three further focus groups were held to feed back and review findings.[14] Nineteen parents, six who had been interviewed individually and 13 who had been part of a focus group, took part. The description and interpretation of the data seemed to be true to their experiences, the additional information from these discussions confirming rather than modifying the analysis.

Results

Fever, cough, and the possibility of meningitis consistently emerged as parents' primary concerns when their children became acutely ill. These provoked particular anxiety because of fears that their child would die or be irreparably harmed. These concerns are

Table 2
Characteristics of participants

	No of households (n=91)
Unemployed household*	34
Living in rented housing	58
Mother left full time education at 16 or under	64
Mother without formal qualifications since leaving school†	54
Single parent household	29
Household with one child	31

*No parent in employment.
†Educational or vocational.

discussed below to illustrate an explanatory scheme of parents' management of ill children developed through the analysis. Two key linked factors were involved: perceived threat and personal control. Other concerns and difficulties parents described are discussed in the accompanying paper.[9]

Perceived threat

Parents' anxieties about fever and cough, and the importance that they attached to them during an episode of illness, related to how parents interpreted their apparent effects on their child. This shaped their assessment of risk or the perceived threat posed by an illness. Of initial concern were changes in behaviour that parents associated with their child becoming unwell, such as not eating or sleeping or not being herself or himself. Parents became more concerned if their child was uncomfortable – for example, hurting from coughing or flushing from fever. They became more anxious if they thought their child was suffering – for example, from the physical effect of a fever or from difficulty in breathing because of coughing (box 1). At this stage parents often worried that the problem might herald more severe illness or potential harm. In the case of fever this included the development of meningitis or fits; permanent impairment of some kind, such as brain

---

Box 1

Suffering and potential harm

Suffering
"I hate it when you see them like that, they're just burning up, lying there crying and not eating" (Parent 11)

"I worry about him getting chesty . . . he really can hardly breathe sometimes he's coughing that much" (Parent 5)

Potential harm
"When their temperature goes too high it's worrying, you worry about brain damage and things, and they could die, or there might be something more deeply worrying than I could imagine" (Parent 20)

Box 2

Managing the problem

"I always keep an eye on the temperature, I Like to get their temperature down, . . . that's the frightening stage when it keeps rising and rising" (Parent 23)

"He sounded like he was choking, I kept making sure he was okay during the night" (Parent 6)

"I panicked and called the doctor . . . she was choking and it was a horrible barking cough and she brought loads of phlegm up making her sick.. there was nothing I could do . . . I thought she was going to die" (Parent 3, group 5)

---

damage; or even death. A fever without other common signs of illness, and therefore an explanation (such as a cold), was especially likely to cause concern and vigilance. For some parents a rising fever posed a more intangible, ill defined threat (box 1).

Coughs that were perceived as "chesty" due to phlegm or that provoked vomiting or retching caused concern about infection "on the chest." Some feared development of a more chronic problem such as asthma or worried about death of their child from the sudden infant death syndrome, from inhaling vomit, or, more usually, from choking. Perceived threat, then, comprised categories reflecting the observed effects of a problem and beliefs about the potential harm that might result (fig 1).

Personal control
Monitoring and maintaining control of symptoms was seen as paramount to minimise discomfort and reduce the threat of harm. Parents continuously assessed their child's temperature (most often by touch) and diligently performed cooling procedures. They were preoccupied with the fever becoming too high: their common fear was of a temperature rising inexorably, eventually spiralling out of their control and bringing the threat of harm nearer. Management of cough entailed a similar process of checking and trying to reduce the effects of the cough,

particularly at night when the child was seen as more vulnerable and difficult to monitor. Parents felt increasingly powerless when their efforts were failing to keep a problem under control and the perceived threat increased (box 2).

Analysis of parents' strategies showed that they watched, checked, and tried to make sense of their child's illness. At the heart of this lay an imperative responsibility to ensure the safety of their child. Parents expressed frustration at feeling ignorant, and they worried about failing to recognise a serious problem, about missing something (box 3). A parent's personal control encompassed her sense of being able to control the observed effects of an illness and to protect her child from potential harm. This was conditioned by her knowledge, beliefs, and experiences and informed her evaluation and management of a problem. Figure 1 depicts a model of the interaction of personal control regulating perceived threat.

The need to share responsibility with others within their lay network or by seeking professional advice could be irresistible when parents were concerned about their child. Some parents felt guilty about bothering their doctor in these circumstances but thought that they had little choice (box 4). These issues were foremost when parents talked about meningitis. Discussion about meningitis was often emotive. Parents' deepest fears of death or handicap befalling their child crystallised in the form of meningitis. There was a common understanding that symptoms could be non-specific and the illness rapidly overwhelming, heightening anxiety about not detecting the disease. For some parents the spectre of meningitis haunted them whenever their child showed

---

Box 3

Lack of control

"If I knew what the problem was I don't think I'd be as worried, it is not knowing that gets to me" (Parent 16)

"When she's got a bug . . . I'm worried that it's some-thing else, and I'm missing something . . . it could be something nasty . . . I don't know" (Parent 4)

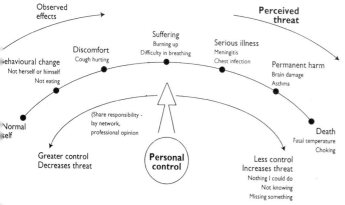

Fig 1—*Interaction of personal control and perceived threat*

Box 4

Sharing responsibility and meningitis fear

Sharing responsibility

Father: "Once the doctor's been out and had a look you feel a lot easier in yourself"

Mother: "You think, 'Am I phoning him up for nothing?' . . . but at the end of the day if you didn't and something happened to your baby you would never forgive yourself" (Parents 15A and B)

Spectre of meningitis

Parent 5: You don't really know what you're looking for do you?

Parent 6: No, I mean you hear about it on the telly and it starts from 'flu symptoms, things like that, and you think straight away they're not getting better, that's it, it must be meningitis

Parent 4: You always worry about meningitis . . . in case you don't catch it quick enough

Parent 5: Well you get no symptoms at the beginning . . . meningitis does not give any warning (Group 3)

---

signs of being more than slightly unwell (box 4). The specific feature of meningitis most often identified was appearance of a rash. Parents were ever vigilant for this sign of meningococcal illness, but few parents had accurate knowledge of the rash. For many parents any unexplained rash could herald immediate danger and the need to seek medical advice.

Discussion

Methodological considerations

This study has highlighted the primary concerns of parents when young children become acutely ill and has explored why they worry about them. A qualitative approach was used to provide insights into parents' concerns and thinking rather than produce statistically representative results. Most parents were willing to participate. I did not gather comprehensive information about non-respondents, however, as I did not want parents to feel uncomfortable or under pressure to participate when many had hectic schedules, particularly in the community centre and toddler groups. Moreover, I wanted a sample of parents who were willing to articulate their experiences.

The systematic methods described were used to increase the reliability and validity of the study: selecting a broad range of parents with different experiences; obtaining data in both one to one and group settings; and reviewing and confirming the findings with participants themselves. In the focus groups parents were already familiar with each other. This may have reduced the artificiality of the discussions. These groups explored one of the social contexts in which ideas might be formed and decisions made about young children's illness. Conversely, respondent validation used

discussions between previously interviewed participants who were not known to each other and allowed comparison of parents' experiences in another context.

Differences between the researcher and respondents may have influenced parents' responses and their interpretation: I am a male middle class health professional and the respondents were largely women from disadvantaged backgrounds. Parents' public accounts may have been selective and excluded that which might be considered unacceptable to a health professional. Participants were aware that I was a doctor, and discussion may have been biased towards medical rather than lay concepts. However, the study has attempted to place emphasis on the perceptions of the parents interviewed. I was also able to identify with some of the respondents' experiences as I have worked as a general practitioner in their community for the past five years. Few fathers were interviewed – the study reflects the contemporary reality of childcare, which remains largely the responsibility of mothers.

Understanding parents' concerns

When parents' concerns were explored, two factors emerged that appeared fundamental in shaping their responses: parents' sense of personal control when faced with illness in their child and the perceived threat posed by an illness. Germane to personal control was parents' experience of comparative ignorance and difficulty in establishing the severity of illness, which is discussed further in the accompanying paper.[9] Parents' concerns were expressed within the context of keenly felt pressure to protect their child from harm. The perceived threat could be seen as a continuous process corresponding to the effects a problem was believed or observed to cause and regulated by a parent's personal control (fig 1). This scheme has resonance with the folk model of illness beliefs proposed by Helman.[15] For example, fever was perceived as serious and its development outside personal control (thus requiring professional advice) in contrast to a common cold, in which the elements of personal responsibility and control are strong, its development being influenced by things such as not wrapping up well.

Parents' concerns about fever and cough reflected erroneous beliefs and use of biomedical concepts, albeit in a rational framework. Beliefs about fever rising relentlessly and the need to control temperature may be viewed as logical and congruent with fairly common knowledge of febrile convulsions and delirium in young children. In addition, advice from professionals commonly reinforces cooling children regularly, particularly in relation to febrile fits. However, controlling temperature is not necessarily preventive – the main purpose is to keep the child comfortable[16] Quantitative research from North America has pointed to similar beliefs.[17 18] Parents may benefit from education about the probable positive effects of fever[19] and the body's central regulatory thermostat.

The depth and nature of parents' concerns about cough accord with the high proportion of consultations

ARTICLE 6

Key messages

- When faced with acute illness in their children, parents' concerns were shaped by their sense of personal control and the perceived threat posed by an illness
- Parents worried about fever, cough, the possibility of meningitis, and failing to recognise a serious problem
- Better understanding of parents' concerns and what causes them may promote more effective communication between health professionals and parents

for children in general practice that are for respiratory illness[1]. Similar beliefs have been described among mothers who recently consulted a general practitioner about their child's cough[20] The qualitative construction of perceived threat in the current study is also consistent with the characteristics of a child's cough which have been found to predict likelihood of consulting a general practitioner.[21] Increasing parents' knowledge of the nature of upper and lower respiratory tract infections and the physiological function of cough in response to infection may be helpful.

Parents' anxieties about meningitis must be interpreted in the light of recent media coverage and campaigns about the illness. The pressure parents experienced may have been intensified by messages such as "knowing the symptoms of meningitis could mean the difference between life and death."[22] Parents readily identified the need to be vigilant for a rash, yet self limiting rashes are common in young children. This may be creating unnecessary anxiety and increased contacts with health services. It underlines the need for information to include good photographs to show how to distinguish the rash of meningococcal illness, such as those in the material produced by Meningitis Research.[23]

Parents' anxieties about failing to recognise a serious illness serve as a reminder that what constitutes common knowledge for doctors may not be readily accessible to parents. Information and education that address parents' concerns may empower parents by influencing perceptions of threat posed by an illness and enhancing personal control. This forms the basis of a hypothesis for further exploration. The findings emphasise the importance of acknowledging and addressing parents' fears and beliefs if a consultation is to help the parent and not be regarded as inappropriate by the health professional. With much current activity in general practice focused on managing the rising demand for out of hours care,[24 25] this research highlights a source of mutual dissatisfaction between the parents of ill young children, who generate much of this workload, and their general practitioners. Better understanding of parents' concerns and what motivates them may promote more effective communication between health professionals and parents.

I thank the parents who took part; Sharon Denley, project secretary; the primary care team of Adelaide Medical Centre for support and encouragement; Ethel Street Surgery, Gladys MacFarlane, Marge Craig, and Karen Gelder for help in recruiting participants; and Pauline Pearson, Ann Crosland, Kevin Jones, Rosie Stacy, John Howie, and an anonymous referee for helpful comments. Funding: Northern and Yorkshire Regional Health Authority.
Conflict of interest: None.

References

[1] McCormick A, Fleming D, Charlton J. *Morbidity statistics from general practice: fourth national study 1991-92.* London: HMSO, 1995.
[2] Wilkin D, Hallam L, Leavey R, Metcalfe D. *Anatomy of urban general practice.* London: Tavistock, 1987.
[3] Campion PD, Gabriel J. Child consultation patterns in general practice: comparing "high" and "low" consulting families. *BMJ* 1984;**288**:1426-8.
[4] Spencer N, Logan S, Scholey S, Gentle S. Deprivation and bronchiolitis. *Arch Dis Child* 1996;**74**:50-2.
[5] Blaxter M, Patterson E. *Mothers and daughters: a three generational study of health attitudes and behaviour.* London: Heinemann, 1982.
[6] Spencer NJ. Parents' recognition of the ill child. In: MacFarlane JA, ed. *Progress in child health.* Edinburgh: Churchill Livingstone, 1984:100-1.
[7] Mayall B. *Keeping children healthy.* London: Allen and Unwin, 1986.
[8] Cunningham-Burley S. Mothers' beliefs about and perceptions of their children's illness. In: Cunningham-Burley S, McKeganey N, eds. *Readings in medical sociology.* London: Routledge, 1990:85-109.
[9] Kai J. Parents' difficulties and information needs in coping with acute illness in preschool children: a qualitative study. *BMJ* 1996;**313**:987-90.
[10] Glaser BG, Strauss AL, *The discovery of grounded theory.* New York: Aldine, 1967.
[11] Bogdan R C, Biklen SR. *Qualitative research for education: an introduction to theory and methods.* Boston: Allyn and Bacon, 1982.
[12] Kreuger R. *Focus groups, a practical guide for applied research.* London: Sage, 1988.
[13] Strauss A, Corbin J. *Basics of qualitative research. Grounded theory procedures and techniques.* London: Sage, 1990.
[14] Mays N, Pope C. Rigour and qualitative research. *BMJ* 1995;**311**:109-12.
[15] Helman C. Feed a cold, starve a fever. In: Currer C, Stacey M, eds. *Concepts of health, illness and disease: a comparative perspective.* Leamington Spa: Berg, 1986.
[16] Stephenson T, Dunn K. The febrile child. *Maternal and Child Health* 1994;**19**:128-32.
[17] Schmitt BD. Fever phobia. *Am J Dis Child* 1980;**134**:176-81.
[18] Kramer MS, Naimark L, Leduc DG. Parental fever phobia and its correlates. *Paediatrics* 1985;**75**:1110-3.
[19] Kluger NJ. The adaptive value of fever. In: Mackowiak PA, ed. *Fever: basic mechanisms and management.* New York: Raven Press, 1991.
[20] Cornford CS, Morgan M, Ridsdale L. Why do mothers consult when their children cough? *Fam Pract* 1993;**10**:193-6.
[21] Wyke S, Hewison J, Russell I. Respiratory illness in children: what makes parents decide to consult? *J R Coll Gen Pract* 1990;**40**:226-9.
[22] Department of Health. *Knowing about meningitis and septicaemia.* London: DoH, 1994. (Leaflet.)
[23] Meningitis Research. *What to do if you suspect meningitis.* Bristol: Meningitis Research, 1994.
[24] Hallam L. Primary medical care outside normal working hours: review of published work. *BMJ* 1994;**308**:249-53.
[25] Hurwitz B. The new out of hours agreement for general practitioners. *BMJ* 1995;**311**:824-5.

(Accepted 7 August 1996)

This article was first published in the BMJ and is reproduced by permission of the BMJ.

This is the fourth of seven articles describing non-quantitative techniques and showing their value in health research

QUALITATIVE INTERVIEWS IN MEDICAL RESEARCH

Nicky Britten

Nicky Britten, *lecturer in medical sociology*

Department of General Practice,
United Medical and Dental Schools of Guy's and St Thomas's Hospitals, London SE11 6SP

BMJ 1995;**311**:251-3

Much qualitative research is interview based, and this paper provides an outline of qualitative interview techniques and their application in medical settings. It explains the rationale for these techniques and shows how they can be used to research kinds of questions that are different from those dealt with by quantitative methods. Different types of qualitative interviews are described, and the way in which they differ from clinical consultations is emphasised. Practical guidance for conducting such interviews is given.

TYPES OF QUALITATIVE INTERVIEW

Practising clinicians routinely interview patients during their clinical work, and they may wonder whether simply talking to people constitutes a legitimate form of research. In sociology and related disciplines, however, interviewing is a well established research technique. There are three main types: structured, semistructured, and in depth interviews (box 1).

Structured interviews consist of administering structured questionnaires, and interviewers are trained to ask questions (mostly fixed choice) in a standardised manner. For example, interviewees might be asked: "Is your health: excellent, good, fair, or poor?" Though qualitative interviews are often described as being unstructured in order to contrast them with this type of formalised quantitative interview, the term "unstructured" is misleading as no interview is completely devoid of structure: if it were, there would be no guarantee that the data gathered would be appropriate to the research question.

Semistructured interviews are conducted on the basis of a loose structure consisting of open ended questions that define the area to be explored, at least initially, and from which the interviewer or interviewee may diverge in order to pursue an idea in more detail. Continuing with the same example, interviewees might initially be asked a series of questions such as: "What do you think good health is?", "How do you consider your own health?", and so on.

In depth interviews are less structured than this, and may cover only one or two issues, but in much greater detail. Such an interview might begin with the

---

Box 1 – Types of interviews

- Structured
  Usually with a structured questionnaire
- Semistructured
  Open ended questions
- Depth
  One or two issues covered in great detail
  Questions are based on what the interviewee says

---

interviewer saying, "This research study is about how people think about their own health. Can you tell me about your own health experiences and what you think of your health?" Further questions from the interviewer would be based on what the interviewee said and would consist mostly of clarification and probing for details.

Clinical and qualitative research interviews have very different purposes. Although the doctor may be willing to see the problem from the patient's perspective, the clinical task is to fit that problem into an appropriate medical category in order to choose an appropriate form of management. The constraints of most consultations are such that any open ended questioning needs to be brought to a conclusion by the doctor within a fairly short time. In a qualitative research interview the aim is to discover the interviewee 5 own framework of meanings and the research task is to avoid imposing the researcher's structures and assumptions as far as possible. The researcher needs to remain open to the possibility that the concepts and variables that emerge may be very different from those that might have been predicted at the outset.

Qualitative interview studies address different questions from those addressed by quantitative research. For example, a quantitative epidemiological approach to the sudden infant death syndrome might measure statistical correlates of national and regional variations in incidence. In a qualitative study Gantley *et al* interviewed mothers of young babies in different ethnic groups to understand their child rearing practices and hence discover possible factors contributing to the low incidence of sudden infant death in Asian populations.[1] A quantitative study of singlehanded general practitioners might compare their prescribing and referral rates, out of hours payments, list sizes, and immunisation and cervical cytology rates with those of general practitioners in partnerships. A recent qualitative study examined the concerns of singlehanded general practitioners during semi-structured interviews and identified the problems perceived by this group of doctors.[2] Qualitative research can also open up different areas of research such as hospital consultants' views of their patients[3] or general practitioners' accounts of uncomfortable prescribing decisions.[4]

CONDUCTING INTERVIEWS

Qualitative interviewers try to be interactive and sensitive to the language and concepts used by the interviewee, and they try to keep the agenda flexible. They aim to go below the surface of the topic being discussed, explore what people say in as much detail as possible, and uncover new areas or ideas that were not anticipated at the outset of the research. It is vital that interviewers check that they have understood respondents' meanings instead of relying on their own assumptions. This is particularly important if there is obvious potential for misunderstanding—for example, when a clinician interviews someone unfamiliar with medical terminology. Clinicians should not assume that interviewees use medical terminology in the same way that they do.

Patton said that good questions in qualitative interviews should be open ended, neutral, sensitive, and clear to the interviewee.[5] He listed six types of questions that can be asked: those based on behaviour or experience, on opinion or value, on feeling, on knowledge, and on sensory experience and those asking about demographic or background details (box 2). It is usually best to start with questions that the interviewee can answer easily and then proceed to more difficult or sensitive topics. Most interviewees are willing to provide the kind of information the researcher wants, but they need to be given clear guidance about the amount of detail required. It is possible to collect data even in stressful circumstances.[6]

The less structured the interview, the less the questions are determined and standardised before the interview occurs. Most qualitative interviewers will have a list of core questions that define the areas to be covered. Unlike quantitative interviews based on highly structured questionnaires, the order in which questions are asked will vary, as will the questions designed to probe the interviewee's meanings. Wordings cannot be standardised because the interviewer will try to use the person's own

vocabulary when framing supplementary questions. Also, during the course of a qualitative study, the interviewer may introduce further questions as he or she becomes more familiar with the topic being discussed.

All qualitative researchers need to consider how they are perceived by interviewees and the effects of characteristics such as class, race, sex, and social distance on the interview. This question becomes more acute if the interviewee knows that the interviewer is also a doctor. An interviewee who is already a patient or likely to become one may wish to please the doctor by giving the responses he or she thinks the doctor wants. It is best not to interview one's own patients for research purposes, but if this cannot be avoided, patients should be given permission to say what they really think, and they should not be corrected if they say things that doctors think are wrong (for example, that antibiotics are a suitable treatment for viral infections).

Interviewers are also likely to be asked questions by interviewees during the course of an interview. The problem with this is that in answering questions, clinical researchers may undo earlier efforts not to impose their own concepts on the interview. If questions are not answered, this may reduce the interviewee's willingness to answer the interviewer's subsequent questions. One solution is to say that such questions can be answered at the end of the interview, although this is not always a satisfactory response.[7]

RESEARCHER AS RESEARCH INSTRUMENT

Qualitative interviews require considerable skill on the part of the interviewer. Experienced doctors may feel that they already possess the necessary skills, and indeed many are transferable. To achieve the transition from consultation to research interview, clinical researchers need to monitor their own interviewing technique, critically appraising tape recordings of their interviews and asking others for their comments. The novice research interviewer needs to notice how directive he or she is being, whether leading questions are being asked, whether cues are picked up or ignored, and whether interviewees are given enough time to explain what they mean. Whyte devised a six point directiveness scale to help novice researchers analyse their own interviewing technique (box 3).[8] The point is not that non-

ARTICLE 7

Box 2 – Types of questions for qualitative interview[5]

- Behaviour or experience
- Opinion or belief
- Feelings
- Knowledge
- Sensory
- Background or demographic

Box 3 – Whyte's directiveness scale for analysing interviewing technique[8]

1 Making encouraging noises
2 Reflecting on remarks made by the informant
3 Probing on the last remark by the informant
4 Probing an idea preceding the last remark by the informant
5 Probing an idea expressed earlier in the interview
6 Introducing a new topic

(1 =least directive, 6=most directive)

Box 4 – Maintaining control of the interview[5]

- Knowing what it is you want to find out
- Asking the right questions to get the information you need
- Giving appropriate verbal and non-verbal feedback

Box 5 – Common pitfalls in interviewing[9]

- Interruptions from outside (telephone, etc)
- Competing distractions (children, etc)
- Stage fright for interviewer or interviewee
- Asking interviewee embarrassing or awkward questions
- Jumping from one subject to another
- Teaching (for example, giving interviewee medical advice)
- Counselling (for example, summarising responses too early)
- Presenting one's own perspective, thus potentially biasing the interview
- Superficial interviews
- Receiving secret information (for example, suicide threats)
- Translators (for example, inaccuracy)

---

directiveness is always best, but that the amount of directiveness should be appropriate. Some informants are more verbose than others, and it is vital that interviewers maintain control of the interview. Patton provided three strategies for maintaining control: knowing the purpose of the interview, asking the right questions to get the information needed, and giving appropriate verbal and non-verbal feedback (box 4).[5]

Some common pitfalls for interviewers that have been identified by Field and Morse include outside interruptions, competing distractions, stage fright, awkward questions, jumping from one subject to another, and the temptation to counsel interviewees (box 5).[9] Awareness of these pitfalls can help the interviewer to develop ways of overcoming them.

RECORDING INTERVIEWS

There are various ways of recording qualitative interviews: notes written at the time, notes written afterwards, and audiotaping. Writing notes at the time can interfere with the process of interviewing, and notes written afterwards are likely to miss out some details. In certain situations, written notes are preferable to audiotaping, but most people will agree to having an interview tape recorded, although it may take them a little while to speak freely in front of a machine. It is vitally important to use good quality equipment which has been tested beforehand and with which the interviewer is familiar. Transcription is an immensely time consuming process, as each hour's worth of interview can take six or seven hours to transcribe, depending on the quality of the tape. The costing of any interview based study should include adequate transcription time.

IDENTIFYING INTERVIEWEES

Sampling strategies are determined by the purpose of the research project.[9] Statistical representativeness is not normally sought in qualitative research (see the paper by Mays and Pope earlier in this series[10]). Similarly, sample sizes are not determined by hard and fast rules, but by other factors such as the depth and duration of the interview and what is feasible for a single interviewer. Large qualitative studies do not often interview more than 50 or 60 people, although there are exceptions.[11] Sociologists conducting research in medical settings often have to negotiate access with great care, although this is unlikely to be a problem for clinicians conducting research in their own place of work. Nevertheless, the researcher still needs to approach the potential interviewee and explain the purpose of the research, emphasising that a refusal will not affect future

treatment. An introductory letter should also explain what is involved and the likely duration of the interview and should give assurances about confidentiality. Interviews should always be conducted at interviewees' convenience, which for people who work during the day will often be in the evening. The setting of an interview affects the content, and it is usually preferable to interview people at home.

CONCLUSION

Qualitative interviewing is a flexible and powerful tool which can open up many new areas for research. It can enable practising clinicians to investigate research questions of immediate relevance to their everyday work, which would otherwise be difficult to investigate. Few researchers would consider embarking on a new research technique without some form of training, and training in research interviewing skills is available from universities and specialist research organisations.

GREE

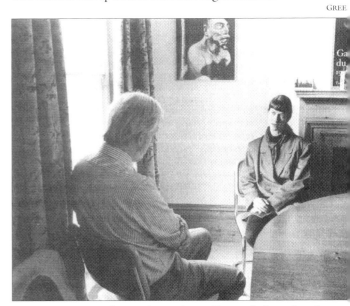

A qualitative research interviewer aims to discover the interviewee's own framework of meanings; the research task is to avoid imposing the researcher's structures and assumptions as far as possible.

Further reading

Fontana A, Frey JH. Interviewing: the art of science. In: Denzin NK, Lincoln YS, eds. *Handbook of qualitative research*. London: Sage, 1994:361-76.

Mishler EG. *Research interviewing: context and narrative*. Cambridge, MA: Harvard University Press, 1986.

References

1. Gantley M, Davies DP, Murcott A. Sudden infant death syndrome: links with infant care practices. *BMJ* 1993;**306**:16-20.
2. Green JM. The views of singlehanded general practitioners: a qualitative study. *BMJ* 1993;**307**:607-10.
3. Britten N. Hospital consultants' views of their patients. *Sociology of Health and Illness* 1991;**13**:83-97.
4. Bradley CP. Uncomfortable prescribing decisions: a critical incident study. *BMJ* 1992;**304**:294-6.
5. Patton MQ. *How to use qualitative methods in evaluation*. London: Sage, 1987:108-43.
6. Cannon S. Social research in stressful settings: difficulties for the sociologist studying the treatment of breast cancer. *Sociology of Health and Illness* 1989;**11**:62-77.
7. Oakley A. Interviewing women: a contradiction in terms. In: Roberts H, ed. *Doing feminist research*. London: Routledge and Kegan Paul, 1981:30-61.
8. Whyte WF. Interviewing in field research. In: Burgess RG, ed. *Field research: a sourcebook and field manual*. London: George Allen and Unwin, 1982: 111-22.
9. Field PA, Morse JM. *Nursing research: the application of qualitative appoaches*. London: Chapman and Hall, 1989.
10. Mays N, Pope C. Rigour and qualitative research. *BMJ;*1995;**311**:109-12.
11. Holland J, Ramazanoglu C, Scott S, Sharpe S, Thomson R. Sex, gender and power: young women's sexuality in the shadow of AIDS. *Sociology of Health and Illness* 1990;**12**:336-50.

ARTICLE 7

This article was first published in the BMJ and is reproduced by permission of the BMJ.

This is the fifth in a series of seven articles describing non-quantitative techniques and showing their value in health research

INTRODUCING FOCUS GROUPS

Jenny Kitzinger

Jenny Kitzinger, *research fellow*

Glasgow University Media Group, Department of Sociology, University of Glasgow, Glasgow G12 8LF

BMJ 1995;**311**:299-302

This paper introduces focus group methodology, gives advice on group composition, running the groups, and analysing the results. Focus groups have advantages for researchers in the field of health and medicine: they do not discriminate against people who cannot read or write and they can encourage participation from people reluctant to be interviewed on their own or who feel they have nothing to say.

RATIONALE AND USES OF FOCUS GROUPS

Focus groups are a form of group interview that capitalises on communication between research participants in order to generate data. Although group interviews are often used simply as a quick and convenient way to collect data from several people simultaneously, focus groups explicitly use group interaction as part of the method. This means that instead of the researcher asking each person to respond to a question in turn, people are encouraged to talk to one another: asking questions, exchanging anecdotes and commenting on each others' experiences and points of view.[1] The method is particularly useful for exploring people's knowledge and experiences and can be used to examine not only what people think but how they think and why they think that way.

Focus groups were originally used within communication studies to explore the effects of films and television programmes,[2] and are a popular method for assessing health education messages and examining public understandings of illness and of health behaviours.[3-7] They are widely used to examine people's experiences of disease and of health services.[8-9] and are an effective technique for exploring the attitudes and needs of staff.[10 11]

The idea behind the focus group method is that group processes can help people to explore and clarify their views in ways that would be less easily accessible in a one to one interview. Group discussion is particularly appropriate when the interviewer has a series of open ended questions and wishes to encourage research participants to explore the issues of importance to them, in their own vocabulary, generating their own questions and pursuing their own priorities. When group dynamics work well the participants work alongside the researcher, taking the research in new and often unexpected directions.

Group work also helps researchers tap into the many different forms of communication that people use in day to day interaction, including jokes, anecdotes, teasing, and arguing. Gaining access to such variety of communication is useful because people's knowledge and attitudes are not entirely encapsulated in reasoned responses to direct questions. Everyday forms of communication may tell us as much, if not more, about what people know or experience. In this sense focus groups reach the parts that other methods cannot reach, revealing dimensions of understanding that often remain untapped by more conventional data collection techniques.

Tapping into such interpersonal communication is also important because this can highlight (sub)cultural values or group norms. Through analysing the operation of humour, consensus, and dissent and examining different types of narrative used within the group, the researcher can identify shared and common knowledge.[12] This makes focus groups a data collection technique particularly sensitive to cultural variables – which is why it is so often used in cross cultural research and work with ethnic minorities. It also makes them useful in studies examining why different sections of the population make differential use of health services.[13 14] For similar reasons focus groups are useful for studying dominant cultural values (for example, exposing dominant narratives about sexuality[15]) and for examining work place cultures – the ways in which, for example, staff cope with working with terminally ill patients or deal with the stresses of an accident and emergency department.

The downside of such group dynamics is that the articulation of group norms may silence individual voices of dissent. The presence of other research

---

Some potential sampling advantages with focus groups

- Do not discriminate against people who cannot read or write
- Can encourage participation from those who are reluctant to be interviewed on their own (such as those intimidated by the formality and isolation of a one to one interview)
- Can encourage contributions from people who feel they have nothing to say or who are deemed "unresponsive patients" (but engage in the discussion generated by other group members)

---

participants also compromises the confidentiality of the research session. For example, in group discussion with old people in long term residential care I found that some residents tried to prevent others from criticising staff – becoming agitated and repeatedly interrupting with cries of "you can't complain"; "the staff couldn't possibly be nicer." On the one hand, such interactions highlighted certain aspects of these people's experiences. In this case, it showed some residents' fear of being "punished" by staff for, in the words of one woman, "being cheeky." On the other hand, such group dynamics raise ethical issues (especially when the work is with "captive" populations) and may limit the usefulness of the data for certain purposes (Scottish Health Feedback, unpublished report).

However, it should not be assumed that groups are, by definition, inhibiting relative to the supposed privacy of an interview situation or that focus groups are inappropriate when researching sensitive topics. Quite the opposite may be true. Group work can actively facilitate the discussion of taboo topics because the less inhibited members of the group break the ice for shyer participants. Participants can also provide mutual support in expressing feelings that are common to their group but which they consider to deviate from mainstream culture (or the assumed culture of the researcher). This is particularly important when researching stigmatised or taboo experiences (for example, bereavement or sexual violence).

Focus group methods are also popular with those conducting action research and those concerned to "empower" research participants because the participants can become an active part of the process of analysis. Indeed, group participants may actually develop particular perspectives as a consequence of talking with other people who have similar experiences. For example, group dynamics can allow for a shift from personal, self blaming psychological explanations ("I'm stupid not to have understood what the doctor was telling me"; "I should have been stronger—I should have asked the right questions") to the exploration of structural solutions ("If we've all felt confused about what we've been told maybe

having a leaflet would help, or what about being able to take away a tape recording of the consultation?").

Some researchers have also noted that group discussions can generate more critical comments than interviews.[16] For example, Geis *et al*, in their study of the lovers of people with AIDS, found that there were more angry comments about the medical community in the group discussions than in the individual interviews: "perhaps the synergism of the group 'kept the anger going' and allowed each participant to reinforce another's vented feelings of frustration and rage."[17] A method that facilitates the expression of criticism and the exploration of different types of solutions is invaluable if the aim of research is to improve services. Such a method is especially appropriate when working with particular disempowered patient populations who are often reluctant to give negative feedback or may feel that any problems result from their own inadequacies.[19]

CONDUCTING A FOCUS GROUP STUDY

Sampling and group composition

Focus group studies can consist of anything between half a dozen to over fifty groups, depending on the aims of the project and the resources available. Most studies involve just a few groups, and some combine this method with other data collection techniques. Focus group discussion of a questionnaire is ideal for testing the phrasing of questions and is also useful in explaining or exploring survey results.[19 20]

Although it may be possible to work with a representative sample of a small population, most focus group studies use a theoretical sampling model (explained earlier in this series[21]) whereby participants are selected to reflect a range of the total study population or to test particular hypotheses. Imaginative sampling is crucial. Most people now recognise class or ethnicity as important variables, and it is also worth considering other variables. For example, when exploring women's experiences of maternity care or cervical smears it may be advisable to include groups of lesbians or women who were sexually abused as children.[22]

Most researchers recommend aiming for homogeneity within each group in order to capitalise on people's shared experiences. However, it can also be advantageous to bring together a diverse group (for example, from a range of professions) to maximise exploration of different perspectives within a group setting. However, it is important to be aware of how hierarchy within the group may affect the data (a nursing auxiliary, for example, is likely to be inhibited by the presence of a consultant from the same hospital).

The groups can be "naturally occurring" (for example, people who work together) or may be drawn together specifically for the research. Using pre-existing groups allows observation of fragments of interactions that approximate to naturally occurring data (such as might have been collected by participant observation). An additional advantage is that friends and colleagues can relate each other's comments to incidents in their shared daily lives. They may challenge each other on contradictions between what they profess to believe and how they actually behave (for example, "how about that time you didn't use a glove while taking blood from a patient?").

It would be naive to assume that group data are by definition "natural" in the sense that such interactions would have occurred without the group being convened for this purpose. Rather than assuming that sessions inevitably reflect everyday interactions (although sometimes they will), the group should be used to encourage people to engage with one another, formulate their ideas, and draw out the cognitive structures which previously have not been articulated.

Finally, it is important to consider the appropriateness of group work for different study populations and to think about how to overcome potential difficulties. Group work can facilitate collecting information from people who cannot read or write. The "safety in numbers factor" may also encourage the participation of those who are wary of an interviewer or who are anxious about talking.[23] However, group work can compound difficulties in communication if each person has a different disability. In the study assessing residential care for the elderly, I conducted a focus group that included one person who had impaired hearing, another with senile dementia, and a third with partial paralysis affecting her speech. This severely restricted interaction between research participants and confirmed some of the staff's predictions about the limitations of group work with this population. However, such problems could be resolved by thinking more carefully about the composition of the group, and sometimes group participants could help to translate for each other. It should also be noted that some of the old people who might have been unable to sustain a one to one interview were able to take part in the group, contributing intermittently. Even some residents who staff had suggested should be excluded from the research because they were "unresponsive" eventually responded to the lively conversations generated by their co-residents and were able to contribute their point of view. Communication difficulties should not rule out group work, but must be considered as a factor.

Running the groups

Sessions should be relaxed: a comfortable setting, refreshments, and sitting round in a circle will help to establish the right atmosphere. The ideal group size is between four and eight people. Sessions may last one to two hours (or extend into a whole afternoon or a

series of meetings). The facilitator should explain that the aim of focus groups is to encourage people to talk to each other rather than to address themselves to the researcher. The researcher may take a back seat at first, allowing for a type of "structured eavesdropping."[24] Later on in the session, however, the researcher can adopt a more interventionist style: urging debate to continue beyond the stage it might otherwise have ended and encouraging the group to discuss the inconsistencies both between participants and within their own thinking. Disagreements within groups can be used to encourage participants to elucidate their point of view and to clarify why they think as they do. Differences between individual one off interviews have to be analysed by the researchers through armchair theorising; differences between members of focus groups should be explored in situ with the help of the research participants.

The facilitator may also use a range of group exercises. A common exercise consists of presenting the group with a series of statements on large cards. The group members are asked collectively to sort these cards into different piles depending on, for example, their degree of agreement or disagreement with that point of view or the importance they assign to that particular aspect of service. For example, I have used such cards to explore public understandings of HIV transmission (placing statements about "types" of people into different risk categories), old people's experiences of residential care (assigning degrees of importance to different statements about the quality of their care), and midwives' views of their professional responsibilities (placing a series of statements about midwives' roles

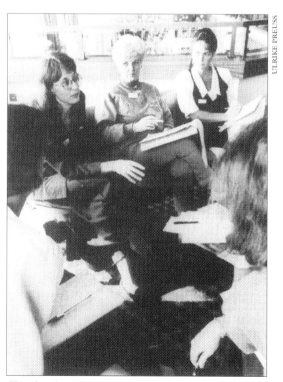

Tapping into interpersonal, communication can highlight cultural values or group norms.

along an agree-disagree continuum). Such exercises encourage participants to concentrate on one another (rather than on the group facilitator) and force them to explain their different perspectives. The final layout of the cards is less important than the discussion that it generates.[25] Researchers may also use such exercises as a way of checking out their own assessment of what has emerged from the group. In this case it is best to take along a series of blank cards and fill them out only towards the end of the session, using statements generated during the course of the discussion. Finally, it may be beneficial to present research participants with a brief questionnaire, or the opportunity to speak to the researcher privately, giving each one the opportunity to record private comments after the group session has been completed.

Ideally the group discussions should be tape recorded and transcribed. If this is not possible then it is vital to take careful notes and researchers may find it useful to involve the group in recording key issues on a flip chart.

Analysis and writing up

Analysing focus groups is basically the same as analysing any other qualitative self report data.[21 26] At the very least, the researcher draws together and compares discussions of similar themes and examines how these relate to the variables within the sample population. In general, it is not appropriate to give percentages in reports of focus group data, and it is important to try to distinguish between individual opinions expressed in spite of the group from the actual group consensus. As in all qualitative analysis, deviant case analysis is important—that is, attention must be given to minority opinions and examples that do not fit with the researcher's overall theory.

The only distinct feature of working with focus group data is the need to indicate the impact of the group dynamic and analyse the sessions in ways that take full advantage of the interaction between research participants. In coding the script of a group discussion, it is worth using special categories for certain types of narrative, such as jokes and anecdotes, and types of interaction, such as "questions," "deferring to the opinion of others," "censorship," or "changes of mind." A focus group research report that is true to its data should also usually include at least some illustrations of the talk between participants, rather than simply presenting isolated quotations taken out of context.

CONCLUSION

This paper has presented the factors to consider when designing or evaluating a focus group study. In particular, it has drawn attention to the overt exploitation and exploration of interactions in focus group discussion. Interaction between participants can be used to achieve seven main aims:

- To highlight the respondents' attitudes, priorities, language, and framework of understanding;
- To encourage research participants to generate and explore their own questions and develop their own analysis of common experiences;
- To encourage a variety of communication from participants—tapping into a wide range and form of understanding;
- To help to identify group norms and cultural values;
- To provide insight into the operation of group social processes in the articulation of knowledge (for example, through the examination of what information is censured or muted within the group);
- To encourage open conversation about embarrassing subjects and to permit the expression of criticism;
- Generally to facilitate the expression of ideas and experiences that might be left underdeveloped in an interview and to illuminate the research participants' perspectives through the debate within the group.

Group data are neither more nor less authentic than data collected by other methods, but focus groups can be the most appropriate method for researching particular types of question. Direct observation may be more appropriate for studies of social roles and formal organisations[27] but focus groups are particularly suited to the study of attitudes and experiences. Interviews may be more appropriate for tapping into individual biographies,[27] but focus groups are more suitable for examining how knowledge, and more importantly, ideas, develop and operate within a given cultural context. Questionnaires are more appropriate for obtaining quantitative information and explaining how many people hold a certain (pre-defined) opinion; focus groups are better for exploring exactly how those opinions are constructed. Thus while surveys repeatedly identify gaps between health knowledge and health behaviour, only qualitative methods, such as focus groups, can actually fill these gaps and explain why these occur.

Focus groups are not an easy option. The data they generate can be as cumbersome as they are complex. Yet the method is basically straightforward and need not be intimidating for either the researcher or the researched. Perhaps the very best way of working out whether or not focus groups might be appropriate in any particular study is to try them out in practice.

Further reading
Morgan D. *Focus groups as qualitative research*. London: Sage, 1988.
Kreuger R. *Focus groups: a practical guide for applied research*. London: Sage, 1988.

References

1. Kitzinger J. The methodology of focus groups: the importance of interactions between research participants. *Sociology of Health and Illness* 1994;**16;** 103-21.

2. Merton R, Fisk M, Kendall P. *The focused interview: a report of the bureau of applied social research.* New York: Columbia University, 1956.

3. Basch C. Focus group interview: an under-utilised research technique for improving theory and practice in health education. *Health Education Quarterly* 1987;**14:**411-8.

4. Kitzinger J. Understanding AIDS: researching audience perceptions of acquired immune deficiency syndrome. In Eldridge I, ed. *Getting the message: news, truth and power.* London: Routledge, 1993:271-305.

5. Ritchie JE, Herscovitch F, Norfor JB. Beliefs of blue collar workers regarding coronary risk behaviours. *Health Education Research* 1994;**9:**95-103.

6. Duke SS, Gordon-Sosby K, Reynolds KD, Gram IT. A study of breast cancer detection practices and beliefs in black women attending public health clinics. *Health Education Research* 1994;**9:**331-42.

7. Khan M, Manderson L. Focus groups in tropical diseases research. *Health Policy and Planning* 1992;**7:**56-66.

8. Murray S, Tapson I, Turnbull L, McCallum J, Little A. Listening to local voices: adapting rapid appraisal to assess health and social needs in general practice. *BMJ* 1994;**308:**698-700.

9. Gregory S, McKie L. The smear test: listening to women's views. *Nursing Standard* 1991;**5:**32-6.

10. Brown J, Lent B, Sas G. Identifying and treating wife abuse. *Journal of Family Practice* 1993;**36:**185-91.

11. Denning JD, Verschelden C. Using the focus group in assessing training needs: empowering child welfare workers. *Child Welfare* 1993;**72:**569-79.

12. Hughes D, Dumont K. Using focus groups to facilitate culturally anchored research. *American Journal of Community Psychology* 1993;**21:**775-806.

13. Zimmerman M, Haffey J, Crane E, Szumowski D, Alvarez F, Bhiromrut P, *et al.* Assessing the acceptability of NORPLANT implants in four countries: findings from focus group research. *Studies in Family Planning* 1990;**21:**92-103.

14. Naish J, Brown J, Denton, B. Intercultural consultations: investigation of factors that deter non-English speaking women from attending their general practitioners for cervical screening. *BMJ* 1994;**309:**1126-8.

15. Barker G, Rich S. Influences on adolescent sexuality in Nigeria and Kenya: findings from recent focus-group discussions. *Studies in Family Planning* 1992;**23:**199-210.

16. Watts M, Ebbutt D. More than the sum of the parts: research methods in group interviewing. *British Educational Research Journal* 1987;**13:**25-34.

17. Geis S, Fuller R, Rush J. Lovers of AIDS victims: psychosocial stresses and counselling needs. *Death Studies* 1986;**10:**43-53.

18. DiMatteo M, Kahn K, Berry S. Narratives of birth and the postpartum: an analysis of the focus group responses of new mothers. *Birth* 1993;**20:**204.

19. Kitzinger J. Focus groups: method or madness?. In Boulton M, ed. *Challenge and innovation: methodological advances in social research on HIV/AIDS.* London: Taylor and Francis, 1994:159-75.

20. O'Brien K. Improving survey questionnaires through focus groups. In Morgan D, ed. *Successful focus groups: advancing the state of the art.* London: Sage, 1993:105-18.

21. Mays N, Pope C. Rigour and qualitative research. *BMJ* 1995;**311:**109-12.

22. Kitzinger J. Recalling the pain: incest survivors' experiences of obstetrics and gynaecology. *Nursing Times* 1990;**86:**38-40.

23. Loderman L. High apprehensives talk about communication apprehension and its effects on their behaviour. *Communication Quarterly* 1983;**31:**233-37.

24. Powney I. Structured eavesdropping. *Research Intelligence (Journal of the British Educational Research Foundation)* 1988;**28:**10-2.

25. Kitzinger J. Audience understanding AIDS: a discussion of methods. *Sociology of Health and Illness* 1990;**12:**319-35.

26. Britten N. Qualitative interviews in medical research. *BMJ* 1995;**311:**251-3.

27. Mays N, Pope C. Observational methods in health care settings. *BMJ* 1995;**311:**182-4.

This article was first published in the BMJ and is reproduced by permission of the BMJ.

This is the third of seven articles describing non-quantitative techniques and showing their value in health research

Observational methods in health care settings

Nicholas Mays, Catherine Pope

Nicholas Mays, *director of health services research* King's Fund, Institute, London W2 4HT

Catherine Pope, *lecturer in social and behavioural medicine* Department of Epidemiology and Public Health, University of Leicester, Leicester LE1 6TP

BMJ 1995;**311**:182-4

Clinicians used to observing individual patients, and epidemiologists trained to observe the course of disease, may be forgiven for misunderstanding the term observational method as used in qualitative research. In contrast to the clinician or epidemiologist, the qualitative researcher systematically watches people and events to find out about behaviours and interactions in natural settings. Observation, in this sense, epitomises the idea of the researcher as the research instrument. It involves "going into the field" – describing and analysing what has been seen. In health care settings this method has been insightful and illuminating, but it is not without pitfalls for the unprepared researcher.

The term "observational methods" seems to be a source of some confusion in medical research circles. Qualitative observational studies are very different from the category of observational studies (non-experimental research designs) used in epidemiology, nor are they like the clinical observation of a patient. Observational methods used in social science involve the systematic, detailed observation of behaviour and talk: watching and recording what people do and say. Goffman neatly captured this distinct research method with his recommendation that, in order to learn about a social group, one should "submit oneself in the company of the members to the daily round of petty contingencies to which they are subject."[1] Thus, observational methods can involve asking questions and analysing documents, but the primary focus on observation makes it distinct from a qualitative research interview (see the next paper in this series) or history taking during patient consultation. Another crucial point about qualitative observation is that it takes place in natural settings not experimental ones; hence, this type of work is often described as "naturalistic research."

RESEARCH ROLES

In an attempt to minimise the impact on the environment being studied the researcher sometimes adopts a "participant observer" role, becoming involved

Box 1 – Observational research roles[2]	
Complete participant	Covert observation
Participant as observer	Overt observation—mutual awareness of the research
Observer as participant	Essentially a one shot interview with no enduring relationship based on lengthy observation
Complete observer	Experimental design, no participation

in the activities taking place while also observing them. The degree of participation varies according to the nature of the setting and the research questions, but broadly corresponds to the first two research roles described in Gold's typology (box 1).[2] There are obviously important ethical considerations about the decision to conduct covert research, and for this reason examples of this type of observational study are rare. However, its use may be justified in some settings, and it has been used to research sensitive topics such as homosexuality[3] and difficult to access areas such as fascist organisations[4] and football hooliganism.[5] Overt research – Gold's "participant as observer" – may pose fewer ethical dilemmas, but this may be offset by the group or individuals reacting to being observed. At its most basic, having a researcher observing actions may stimulate modifications in behaviour or action – the so-called "Hawthorne effect,"[6] or encourage introspection or self questioning among those being researched. In his classic study of street gangs in the United States, Whyte recounted how a key group member said, "You've slowed me up plenty since you've been down here. Now when I do something I have to think what Bill Whyte would want to know about it and how I can explain it. Before I used to do things by instinct."[7]

In addition to these potential problems for the subjects of observational research, there are important considerations for researchers "entering the field." In essence these involve "getting in and getting out." In the initial phases there may be problems gaining access

ARTICLE 9

to a setting, and then in striking up sufficient rapport and empathy with the group to enable research to be conducted. In medical settings, such as a hospital ward, this may involve negotiating with several different staff groups ranging from consultants and junior doctors, to nurse managers, staff nurses, social workers, and auxiliary professions. Once "inside" there is the problem of avoiding "going native"; that is, becoming so immersed in the group culture that the research agenda is lost, or that it becomes extremely difficult or emotionally draining to exit the field and conclude the data collection.

WHAT CAN OBSERVATION TELL US THAT OTHER METHODS CANNOT?

Given these difficulties, observational methods may seem a peculiar choice for studying health and health services. However, an important advantage of observation is that it can help to overcome the discrepancy between what people say and what they actually do. It circumvents the biases inherent in the accounts people give of their actions caused by factors such as the wish to present themselves in a good light, differences in recall, selectivity, and the influences of the roles they occupy. For these reasons, observational methods are particularly well suited to the study of the working of organisations and how the people within them perform their functions. It may also uncover behaviours or routines of which the participants themselves may be unaware. For example, Jeffery's observation of casualty wards in Edinburgh indicated that, because of the conflicting demands and pressures on staff, some patients, who were seen as inappropriate attenders, were labelled as "normal rubbish" and treated differently from "good" patients, who were viewed as more deserving.[8] A similar picture emerges from Hughes's work on the decisions made by reception clerks when patients present themselves at casualty department.[9] It is unlikely that interviews alone would have elicited these different patterns of care. Indeed the labelling of certain cases as "normal rubbish" may have been so embedded in the culture of the casualty setting that only an outsider or newcomer to the scene would have considered it noteworthy.

Another observational study provides an example of how qualitative work can build on existing quantitative research.[10] Against the background of large variations in rates of common surgical procedures such as hysterectomy, cholecystectomy, and tonsillectomy, Bloor observed ear, nose, and throat outpatient clinics to see how decisions to admit children for surgery were made. He systematically analysed how surgeons made their decisions to operate and discovered that individual doctors had different "rules of thumb" for coming to a decision. While one surgeon might take clinical signs as the chief indication for surgery, another might be prepared to operate in the absence of such indications at the time of consultation if there was evidence that repeated episodes of tonsillitis were severely affecting, a

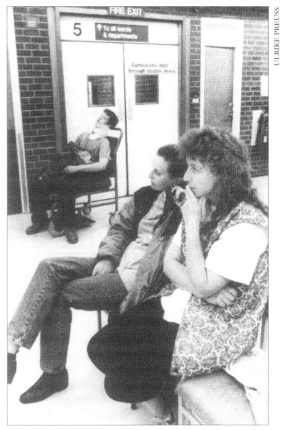

Observation of transactions with patients presenting to casualty departments found that staff classified patients into "normal rubbish" (the inappropriate attenders) and "good" patients, who were viewed as more deserving.

child's education. Understanding the behaviour of these surgeons, knowing why they made their decisions, provided considerable insight into how the variation in surgical rates occurred.

Similar variation and patterning occurs in the statistics on inpatient waiting lists: some surgeons have long lists, others do not; some specialties have long waits, others do not. An observational study showed that rules and routines akin to those discovered by Bloor could be discerned in the day to day management of waiting lists.[11] Surgical and administrative preferences were important in deciding who came off the list. Different reasons for admitting a patient might range from case mix demands for teaching juniors, through ensuring a balanced list, to the ease with which a patient could be contacted and offered admission. Thus, observing how waiting lists work can indicate which policy and administrative changes are likely to have an impact in reducing lists and which are not: a policy which assumed that waiting lists operated as first come, first served queues would be unlikely to affect the day to day routines described above.

SOME RULES ABOUT OBSERVATION
Sampling
Before any recording and analysis can take place, the Setting to be observed has to be chosen. As in other qualitative research, this sampling is seldom

ARTICLE 9

statistically based. Instead, it is likely to be purposive, whereby the researcher deliberately samples a particular group or setting (see Mays and Pope[12] in this series for more on this). The idea of this type of sampling is not to generalise to the whole population but to indicate common links or categories shared between the setting observed and others like it. At its most powerful, the single case can demonstrate features or provide categories relevant to a wide number of settings. Goffman's observation of mental hospitals in the 1960s generated the valuable concept of the "total institution," of which the asylum was one example alongside others such as prisons and monasteries.[1]

Recording

Qualitative observation involves watching and recording what people say and do. As it is impossible to record everything, this process is inevitably selective and relies heavily on the researcher to act as the research instrument and document the world he or she observes. Therefore it is vital that the observations are systematically recorded and analysed, either through the traditional medium of field notes written during or immediately after the events occur or by using audio or video recording facilities. From his unique position as a patient in a tuberculosis sanatorium, Roth was able to record events as they happened,[13] but such situations are rare and most researchers, whether in covert or more participative roles, find that recording necessitates the development of memory skills and frequent trips to the lavatory to "writeup."

The systematic recording of data in qualitative observation distinguishes it from other types of observation such as a tourist recording with a camcorder or a nosey neighbour peering over the fence. Even with video and sound recording it is impossible to "get everything," but as far as possible the researcher aims to record exactly what happened, including his or her own feelings and responses to the situations witnessed. The subjective nature of this type of research contrasts with the objective stance aspired to in the experimental method, but in fact it is a crucial component of the process of analysing qualitative observational data. The researcher usually keeps a field diary or record of the research process to detail events, personal reactions to events, and changes in his or her views over time. Frequently this is the basis of tentative hypotheses or the evolution of systems of classification. In developing classifications or hypotheses it is particularly important to detail any contradictory or negative cases – the unusual, out of the ordinary things which often reveal most about the setting or situation. Tentative classifications and the search for negative cases during the data collection are important facets of the analytic technique used in observational research.

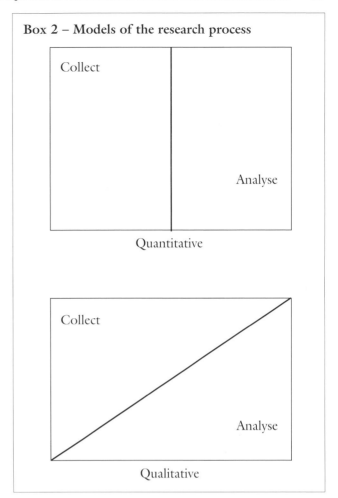

Box 2 – Models of the research process

Collect / Analyse — Quantitative

Collect / Analyse — Qualitative

Analysis

The fieldnotes gathered during observational research are likely to be detailed, highly descriptive accounts and are therefore cumbersome. As descriptions alone they cannot provide explanations. The researcher's task is to sift and decode the data to make sense of the situation, events, and interactions observed. Often this analytical process starts during the data collection phase, a quite different model of the research process to that found in quantitative research, where data collection is completed before any analysis begins (box 2).

Just as the data are systematically recorded, so they are also systematically analysed. Various ways of dealing with observational data have been described, including "analytic induction" and "constant comparison."[14] Stripped of their theoretical trappings, these methods are all variants of content analysis and involve an iterative process of developing categories from the transcripts or fieldnotes, testing them against hypotheses, and refining them. This analytical process is described in detail by Bloor, based on the observational study of ear, nose, and throat clinics described earlier (box 3).[15]

As with quantitative work, it is important that evidence from the data is presented to support the conclusions reached. This can take the form of examples of specific cases, descriptions of events, or quotations. The validity of observational accounts relies on the truthful and systematic representation of the research; in

Box 3 – Analysis

Stages in the analysis of field notes in a qualitative study of ear, nose, and throat surgeons' disposal decisions for children referred for possible tonsillectomy and adenoidectomy (T&A)[11]

(1) Provisional classification—For each surgeon all cases categorised according to the disposal category used (for example, T&A or tonsillectomy alone)

(2) Identification of provisional case features – Common features of cases in each disposal category identified (for example, most T&A cases found to have three main clinical signs present)

(3) Scrutiny of deviant cases – Include in (2) or modify (1) to accommodate deviant cases (for example, T&A performed when only two of three signs present)

(4) Identification of shared case features – Features common to other disposal categories (history of several episodes of tonsillitis, for example)

(5) Derivation of surgeons' decision rules – From the common case features (for example, case history more important than physical examination)

(6) Derivation of surgeons' search procedures (for each decision rule)—The particular clinical signs looked for by each surgeon

Repeat (2) to (6) for each disposal category

many ways it is honesty which separates the observational account from a novel. Hughes says that observational studies should communicate the culture and rules of the setting well enough to allow another researcher to learn them and "pass" as a member of the group.[16] This is not an easy task, and observational research is therefore particularly demanding of the individual researcher.

This brief review has indicated how observational methods can be used to "reach the parts that other methods cannot." Done well, there is no reason why observation should not be as systematic, rigorous, or valid as other research styles and deserve its place in the health researcher's methodological tool box.

Further reading:

Fielding N. *Researching social life*. London: Sage, 1993.

References

1. Goffman E. *Asylums*. Harmondsworth: Penguin, 1961.
2. Gold R. Roles in sociological field investigation. *Social Forces* 1958;**36**:217-23.
3. Humphreys L. *Tearoom trade: impersonal sex in public places*. Chicago: Aldine, 1970.
4. Fielding N. *The National Front*. London: Routledge and Kegan Paul, 1981.
5. Pearson G. *Hooligan: a history of respectable fears*. London: Macmillan, 1983.
6. Roethlisberger FJ, Dickson WI. *Management and the worker*. Cambridge, MA: Harvard University Press, 1939.
7. Whyte WF. *Street corner society: the social structure of an Italian slum*. Chicago: Chicago University Press, 1955.
8. Jeffery R. Normal rubbish: deviant patients in casualty departments. *Sociology of Health and Illness* 1979;**1**:90-108.
9. Hughes D. Paper and people: the work of the casualty reception clerk. *Sociology of Health and Illness* 1990;**11**:382-408.
10. Bloor M. Bishop Berkeley and the adenotonsillectomy enigma: an exploration of the social construction of medical disposals. *Sociology* 1976;**10**:43-61.
11. Pope C. Trouble in store: some thoughts on the management of waiting lists. *Sociology of Health and Illness* 1991;**13**:193-212.
12. Mays N, Pope C. Rigour in qualitative research. *BMJ* 1995;**311**:109-12.
13. Roth J. *Timetables: structuring the passage of time in hospital treatment and other careers*. New York: Bobbs Merrill, 1963.
14. Bryman A, Burgess R, eds. *Analysing qualitative data*. London: Routledge, 1993.
15. Bloor M. On the analysis of observational data: a discussion of the worth and uses of inductive techniques and respondent validation. *Sociology* 1978;**12**:545-52.
16. Hughes I. *Sociological analysis: methods of discovery*. London: Nelson, 1976.

This article was first published in Quality in Health Care and is reproduced by permission of the BMJ Publishing Group.

QUALITATIVE METHODS FOR ASSESSING HEALTH CARE

Ray Fitzpatrick, Mary Boulton

Ray Fitzpatrick, fellow, **Nuffield College, Oxford OX1 1NF**

Mary Boulton, senior lecturer, **Academic Department of Public Health, St Mary's Hospital Medical School, London W2 1PG**

Correspondence to: Dr Fitzpatrick

Quality in Health Care 1994;**3**:107–113

The evaluation of health care and efforts to maintain and improve quality in health care have very largely drawn on quantitative methods. Quantification has made possible precise expression of the extent to which interventions are efficient, effective, or appropriate and has allowed the use of statistical techniques to assess the significance of findings. For many questions, however, quantitative methods may be neither feasible nor desirable. Qualitative methods may be more appropriate when investigators are "opening up" a new field of study or are primarily concerned to identify and conceptualise salient issues. Various qualitative methods have been developed which potentially have an enormous role in assessing health care. This paper examines some of the more important forms that have been used in that assessment and outlines principles of good practice in the application of qualitative methodology. It is intended to encourage a wider use of qualitative methods in assessing health care and a greater appreciation of how much such methods have to offer.

The term "qualitative" is sometimes used quite loosely. We will review some of the methods to which the term is properly applied, but first what is *not* a qualitative study should be emphasised. Research based on a small number of patients or respondents should not be considered qualitative just because the sample size is too small to assess statistical significance. This is more likely to prove to be an inadequate quantitative study. Similarly, a study is not qualitative because it is based on answers to a questionnaire about subjective matters nor because data are collected by personal interview. If such data are analysed and reported largely in terms of frequencies and proportions of respondents expressing particular views, that is also a quantitative study. Qualitative research depends upon not numerical but *conceptual* analysis and presentation. It is used where it is important to understand the meaning and interpretation of human social arrangements such as hospitals, clinics, forms of management, or decision making. Qualitative methods are intended to convey to policy makers the experiences of individuals, groups, and organisations who may be affected by policies.

QUALITATIVE METHODS OF DATA COLLECTION

Qualitative methods of collecting data encompass a range of approaches.

Qualitative methods of data collection
- In depth interviews
- Focus groups
- Nominal group techniques
- Observational studies
- Case studies

In depth interviews

Perhaps the main method of obtaining data for qualitative analysis is by interview. Interviews are a particularly flexible method of gathering data, allowing the investigator to respond to the individual way in which respondents interpret and answer questions. There are various interview formats, but qualitative analysis requires "in depth" interviews so the interviewer can obtain more detailed information than is possible, for example, from an interviewer administered questionnaire, particularly regarding the perceptions and reasons behind respondents' statements. Interviews may be "semistructured," where the interviewer has a fixed set of topics to discuss, or "unstructured," where the interviewer has only very broad objectives in relation to the interview and is largely led by the respondent's priorities and concerns. Unstructured interviews are most appropriate when subject matter is particularly complex or when investigators want to understand reasons for views or are exploring areas which have not previously been extensively described. An interview format increasingly used in health services research is the "critical incident technique," in which respondents are asked to recall the details of a particular experience such as hospitalisation.[1]

Because in depth interviews require the active participation and judgement of the interviewer it is important that they be conducted by interviewers who

ARTICLE 10

have been appropriately trained. There is a range of general interviewing skills that are relevant to performance, such as an ability to demonstrate interest in the respondent without excessive involvement that may result in bias and an ability to ask both open ended facilitating questions and specific probes when relevant. The interviewer also needs to understand the general objectives of a study as well as the intentions behind specific questions. Another essential requirement is that interviewers be perceived by respondents as neutral with regard to the subject matter of an interview. For example, hospital staff are inappropriate to conduct interviews about patient satisfaction, and individuals perceived as judgemental are inappropriate for more sensitive topics.

The analysis of in depth interviews normally entails some degree of formal content analysis of what the respondent has said. For this reason investigators usually tape record interviews which can then be transcribed for detailed content analysis. Broad principles of content analysis for qualitative research are discussed below as, to some extent, they are common to all of the methods discussed in this paper.

An illustration of the use of in depth interviews is a study of the neurological management of chronic headache.[2,3] Neurologists were unsure about the appropriateness of their role in this area. The initial purpose of the study was to identify the expectations of patients with chronic headache regarding their neurological referral, and to establish whether those expectations were satisfied. When interviewed before their outpatient appointments, patients proved quite unsure what to expect. Content analysis of these interviews instead disclosed a small number of different concerns felt by patients about their headaches – for example, a need to be reassured about serious disease or a desire to receive advice about how to change lifestyle or diet to avoid headaches. After their neurological consultations a minority of patients did experience serious disappointment with their clinic attendance but for various reasons were very uncomfortable with the language of "satisfaction" or "dissatisfaction" to describe their experiences. Overall the study suggested particular failures of communication in clinics that led to some patients' concerns not being fully addressed.

In this example the primary advantage of in depth interviews was that they allowed the investigator to focus maximally on patients' perceptions of their health problems and responses to health care rather than imposing his own categories. This led to a new and more meaningful typology of patients' concerns. Examples of other qualitative analyses of in depth interviews include studies of dimensions of patients' experiences of care for various chronic health problems,[4] of the role of clinical audit in British medicine,[5] of informal reasons for clinicians' use of echocardiography,[6] and of the concerns of singlehanded GPs in an inner London area.[7]

Focus groups

Groups rather than individuals may be interviewed by means of a technique commonly referred to as a focus group. Typically, eight to ten individuals are recruited to a group discussion about specified topics. The discussion is led by a trained moderator or facilitator and normally lasts for one and a half to two hours. The discussion is tape recorded, transcribed, and subjected to content analysis. Rather like the interviewer conducting in depth interviews, the moderator has a clear agenda of issues on which he or she stimulates discussion but aims to be fairly non-directive in encouraging discussion. Membership of a focus group needs to be reasonably homogeneous, too much heterogeneity in terms of social background or perspective on a topic tends to result in participants feeling inhibited from revealing views. Therefore if the purpose is to identify the range of views of individuals of different social backgrounds the normal practice is to conduct a series of focus groups.

Focus groups are particularly useful where investigators wish to establish quickly the range of perspectives on an issue of importance among different groups for example, when it is felt necessary to "bridge a gulf" in understanding between providers of a service and the intended users. The dynamics of a well conducted focus group are such that individuals' revelations of their views can "spark off" other participants to reveal broader insights than are possible from individual interviews. However, focus group methods have been compared to "pulling teeth" to stimulate discussion in a group that has no experience or interest in a topic.[8] It is less appropriate in a focus group to probe for elaboration of individuals' statements than is possible in an in depth interview, so that focus groups may be said to be stronger on breadth than depth. The facilitator is less in control of a focus group than is an interviewer with single respondents so it is a method that maximises the expression of perspectives not imposed by the researchers. There are some topics that are sufficiently sensitive that group discussion is inhibiting whereas individual interviews provide a more confidential context for self revelation.

Focus groups are commonly regarded as an exploratory method, so that investigators may conduct them in order to design the questionnaire for a more definitive quantitative survey. Some would argue, however, that focus groups can provide valuable evidence in their own right, provided that investigators are concerned with conceptual rather than numerical analysis.[9]

There are questions still to be addressed with focus group methodology. For example, little is known about how the effects of social desirability and conformity influence expression of views and to what extent heterogeneity of participants influences results. Similarly, though facilitators clearly require substantial interpersonal skills such as ability to listen and to facilitate without becoming so involved as to bias discussion, facilitator effects on the quality of focus groups are not well understood.[9] However, health is a particularly appropriate application for this method,[10] which is being increasingly advocated for use by purchasers in obtaining local views about health and health care.[11, 12]

Nominal group techniques

For some purposes a more impersonal and less threatening form of group dynamics may be needed. A somewhat more structured form of gathering data from groups has been developed, called "nominal groups" because exchange and interaction between group members is more controlled than in focus groups. It is considered a technique less prone to the bias arising from vocal individuals influencing a group's views in open discussion.[13]

A nominal group normally is composed of eight members who meet together with a leader who introduces the group's tasks. The leader explains the question or problem on which the group's views are sought. Individuals are asked to list on a paper form their different feelings or experiences in relation to the question (for example, different kinds of disappointments experienced by a group of users of a clinic), without discussion with other group members. Participants are then asked to declare their written comments which are recorded, as closely as possible to the participants' own words, on a blackboard or flipchart. The complete list is then discussed by the group and a preliminary ranking made by the group from most to least important item of the total list. After discussion of this preliminary ranking a second, private ranking of items is performed by individuals on paper. This information constitutes the researcher's core data. As with focus groups, investigators usually set up several different groups that are needed to represent the different perspectives with interests involved with an issue.

The primary advantages of this form of group research are that individuals may give more carefully considered expressions of their views compared with focus groups and are constrained by the tasks to produce more structured and explicit priorities. The structured nature of data gathering means that this is a method particularly appropriate to contexts where technical or complex issues need to be assessed. The primary disadvantage is that individuals are discouraged from "sparking off" each other, so that it is possible that the full range of views and observations are not elicited. Overall, like focus groups, nominal group techniques are a relatively low cost and quick method of exploring the parameters of an issue.

A variant of this methodology has been developed for use in developing professional consensus about appropriate indications for health care interventions. Panels representing relevant clinical expertise are provided with patient vignettes with varying symptoms and other indications. Vingettes are privately rated in terms of degree of appropriateness for the intervention. The group is then actually assembled, it discusses the ratings, and it is given the opportunity to revise prior decisions. A recent example indicates that substantial agreement could be obtained regarding appropriateness for prostatectomy.[14] Most of the steps in data gathering and interpretation of this application of nominal group techniques are actually quantitative, and readers are referred elsewhere for methodological problems associated with such techniques.[15]

Observational studies

When the research question concerns what actually happens in health care settings, rather than participants' perceptions of and responses to it, a more appropriate method of data collection may be direct observation. For this method the investigators attend the events they are concerned with, pay close attention to what goes on, and make a careful record of it for future analysis, using analytical techniques similar to those for other qualitative data.

Careful recording of what occurs is the cornerstone of observational research. Field notes, taken during or immediately after periods of observation, have been the traditional method of recording. The value of field notes depends on the skill and discipline of the investigator in recording as much detail as accurately as possible. Field notes are inevitably selective and so may be subject to observer bias. However, they are a relatively efficient way of recording observations, particularly in sensitive situations, and provide data in a form that is immediately accessible for analysis. Audio recordings and video recordings provide a more detailed and accurate record of events, although the demands of the technology may limit the range of events that can be observed and the tapes themselves present considerable additional demands in terms in transcription before analysis. Tape recordings are attractive in that they allow the investigator to go back and "reobserve" events, which may allow more detailed analysis than is possible with field notes. They also afford a record of the evidence on which interpretations are made which may be inspected by independent observers in establishing the validity of the analysis. However, audio recorders and particularly video recorders have been criticised as being so obtrusive as to change the nature of the events they are recording, thereby invalidating the observation itself. With smaller machines and consulting rooms specifically adapted for recording this is becoming less of a problem, and, in any case, those who have been the subject of audio or video recording have almost always found that the need to deal with the immediate demands of the situation constrain them to carry on in such the same way as they would if they were not being observed.

Investigators may collect data as "participant" or as "non-participant observers." Participant observers participate in the daily life of the organisation over an extended period of time, watching what happens, listening to what is said, and asking questions. It is an exceptionally demanding way of gathering data. The researcher may encounter difficulties in being accepted by the group initially and then in sustaining the role long enough to observe the full range of events. The justification for such efforts is in the way participant observation enables the researcher to see and experience the institutional culture from the point of view of an "insider." Goffman's classic study of asylums illustrates well the unique insights that can be gained by this method of data collection.[16] Goffman joined an American mental hospital as the assistant to the athletic director in order to observe the culture of the institution without drawing attention to himself. The resulting study develops the concept of the "total institution," identifying its core elements and using it as a framework to describe and make sense of the culture of both the patients and the staff. By closely examining what actually went on in the hospital, he was able to get behind official accounts of what the institution did to show the process and strategies that made it work in practice, and the consequences they had for patients' lives.

Participant observation has become less common as a research method, partly because of questions raised about the ethics of covert observation. Non-participant observation allows the researcher to remain as an accepted outsider, watching and recording the interactions as a "fly on the wall." Non-participant observation is particularly useful when the researcher is concerned to describe and conceptualise the "taken for granted" practices of everyday medical life: the routines and strategies that those they are studying develop in carrying out their work which may be so common and familiar as to be outside their conscious awareness. An example is Strong's study described in *The Ceremonial Order of the Clinic* in which he set out to elucidate the rules which govern interactions in medical consultations.[17] On the basis of observations of 1120 paediatric consultations in several medical settings in Scotland and the United States he documented in detail the existence, nature, and scope of the rules which make up the limited number of institutionalised roles universally adopted by patients and doctors.

The main advantage of observation as a method of data collection is in allowing the investigators to "see for themselves," thus avoiding the biases inherent in participants' reports, such as selective perception, poor recall, and the desire to present themselves well. It is particularly appropriate when the investigator is concerned with describing and conceptualising how health services operate – that is, with practices and processes which are directly accessible to an outside observer. Its main drawback is that it limits the number and range of situations that can be studied to those at which the investigator is present. It is the most labour intensive form of data collection and perhaps for this reason is more often used in conjunction with other methods rather than as the main source of data.

Case studies

Case studies are not really a distinctive method of data collection or analysis but warrant separate discussion because they are increasingly used in the study of health care systems. They provide interpretations and analyses that are ultimately qualitative in nature. The most

obvious respect in which case studies are qualitative is that typically they involve the study of a single or small number of units where quantitative manipulation of variables associated with units would be inappropriate. However, to a greater extent than the methods discussed so far, case studies often draw on mixture of quantitative and qualitative data. An example illustrates the point. In 1986 a resource management (RM) initiative was announced for the NHS, the purpose of which was to improve patient care by providing systems whereby managers and clinicians made better informed and more effective use of resources. The initiative was to be piloted in six acute hospitals and the costs and benefits were to be evaluated by a research team.[18] Much quantitative data were gathered by investigators in relation to hospital activities and their costs in the pilot sites over time. However, as a number of other institutional changes to the NHS were simultaneously having effects in both the study hospitals and any potential "control" hospitals outside the pilot it was decided that it would be impossible to isolate quantitative benefits due to the resource management initiative specifically. Moreover, as with most human organisations, NHS defined objectives of the resource management inititative drifted over time. The authors concluded that qualitative evaluation of the initiative base on qualitative and quantitative evidence available was more informative. Qualitative inferences were drawn from the study such as that it was possible to involve clinicians in hospital resource management but that it was not clear that the high administrative and other costs associated with such involvement were matched by benefits to patient care.

Case studies such as the resource management study usually entail a combination of methods. Investigators carry out interviews, conduct participant observation on relevant meetings, and inspect written documents such as minutes or records. A systematic approach to interviews in an organisation can be adopted. For example, in a study of the impact of general management in the NHS, investigators, if confronted with discrepant accounts between different actors, would probe in interviews to obtain possible explanations.[19] Case studies attempt to get an accurate picture by means of "triangulation," whereby the degree of convergence between different sources (for example, interview and documents) is carefully considered.[20] A particular form of checking the plausibility of investigators' explanations is that of 'respondent validation' in which the analysis that has emerged of a setting is presented to participants for their reactions. By means of this technique analysis can be refined and improved by respondents' feedback.[19]

QUALITATIVE ANALYSIS OF DATA

If the distinguishing feature of quantitative evidence is the manipulation of numerical data then qualitative analysis is characterised by the development and manipulation of *concepts*. The investigator's primary tasks are the inspection and coding of his or her data in terms of concepts and then the manipulation of such concepts into analyses of

. . . qualitative analysis is characterised by the development and manipulation of concepts.

underlying patterns. Although there are significant differences of form or emphasis, this crucial role of conceptual analysis is common to all of the qualitative methods outlined above. It is probably the phase of work that is most arcane and mysterious for audiences of qualitative reports and requires some account of how conceptual analysis of qualitative data is actually done.

Whatever method of data collection is used in qualitative methodology, it results in raw material in the form of "text" – written words. The first stage of processing text is to code and classify. The investigator therefore reviews his or her textual material for coding in terms of concepts and categories that may emerge from the material or that inform the investigator's study to begin with. This transformed, coded material can then be regrouped or indexed to facilitate further analysis. This stage of grouping and indexing coded material has been considerably eased by the development of computer packages such as Ethnograph, although such technology cannot replace the far more important human interpretation of text before mechanical manipulation.[21]

The next and most difficult stage is the analysis of both the original textual data and the transformed conceptual material. This phase is the most difficult to prescribe or indeed describe since it entails a large amount of creative interpretation of evidence. Thought processes include constant comparison of evidence regarding different settings or viewpoints represented in the data and the search for deviant or contrasting observations. One very common feature of this central analytical phase is the development of typologies that convey the range of views, responses, or arrangements under study. Indeed a typology may be one of the central results of a qualitative analysis. Thus in the example cited earlier of a study of patients presenting headaches to neurological clinics a key insight into the strengths and weaknesses of such clinics came from developing a typology of the different major concerns that motivated patients to seek medical help for headache. Patients' views of the benefits of such clinics could be largely understood in terms of these different concerns. A quite contrasting study analysing the role of medical audit advisory groups (MAAGs) identified a typology of three different major models of MAAG.[22] Often it is simply that certain unanticipated themes emerge from content analysis. Elsewhere in this issue (p 69) is described an important study of stroke survivors' views of the benefits of physiotherapy.[23] Several patients regarded physiotherapy as a source of faith and hope for the future. The authors argue that such insights would not emerge from the current batteries of available patient satisfaction instruments used in quantitative

analysis, which concentrate on more familiar dimensions of process and outcome.

A variety of intimidating terms have been developed to describe the logic of qualitative analysis including "analytic induction" and "grounded theory"[24] In different ways such accounts emphasise one common feature – namely, that qualitative analysis is iterative. The investigator goes back and forth between his developing concepts and ideas and the raw data of texts or, ideally, fresh observations of the field.

GOOD PRACTICE FOR QUALITATIVE RESEARCH

The accusation is sometimes made that qualitative research is an "easy option." This usually takes the form of an invidious contrast between informally acquired impressions and the systematic rigour of quantitative methodology. In reality the difficulties of obtaining and conveying insights that are convincing to relevant audiences are at least as great for qualitative research. This section outlines some of the general principles of good practice for qualitative methods that have been developed to facilitate analyses that are plausible and relevant to policy (box). These principles are further developed in a growing number of more detailed guides to qualitative methodology.[25-27]

Principles of good practice for qualitative research

- Theoretical sampling
- Validation
- Conceptual analysis

Sampling

In quantitative studies considerable attention is given to obtaining a sample which is statistically representative of the population of interest so that generalisations may be made from the study. This is generally achieved through random sampling. In qualitative studies numerical generalisations are less important than *conceptual* generalisations. In this case what it is important in drawing a sample is to ensure that it contains the full *range* of possible observations so that the concepts and categories developed provide a comprehensive conceptualisation of the subject. The way in which this is done is through "theoretical sampling."[28] On the basis of his or her theoretical understanding the investigator determines what factors might affect variability in the observations and then endeavours to draw the sample in a way which maximises the variability. This may be decided in advance so that, for example, in a study of a clinic the investigator may be careful to interview patients of varying age, sex, social class, and ethnic background or patients seen by different doctors at different times of day. Theoretical sampling may also require adjusting sources of observation in the course of a study to respond to unanticipated patterns or subgroups of experience which may need increased representation in the sample.

Because qualitative data are more cumbersome to manipulate and analyse most qualitative studies are restricted to a small sample size which is unlikely to be statistically representative of the population. Nevertheless, accounts of qualitative research should always provide a clear account of sampling strategies to allow readers to judge the generalisability the conceptual analyses.

Validity

In the same way every effort is required to establish the validity of analyses based on qualitative material. The two most commonly cited methods of validating qualitative analysis have already been mentioned in relation to case studies - that is, triangulation and respondent validation. In the first method every effort is made to obtain evidence from as diverse and independent a range of sources as possible. This approach is not very different from the process of establishing construct validity for quantitative measures in that one is looking for patterns of convergence between data sources that together corroborate an overall interpretation. Respondent validation requires that investigators obtain subjects' reactions to their analysis and incorporate such reactions into a more complete analysis. However, neither method provides a perfect solution to the problem of validation. Unfortunately, establishing the plausibility of analyses of social settings and organisations such as health care cannot be done by mechanical use of procedures such as triangulation or respondent validation. The world of health care is particularly complex and interpretations of decisions, behaviour, and arrangements will generally vary among participants. Participants may have various reasons for not agreeing with analyses of their behaviour, and, indeed, such disagreements may provide further revealing evidence of how an organisation works.[26]

It is therefore important that users of qualitative methods adopt a number of principles to convince audiences of the validity of their analyses. Have investigators sampled the diverse range of individuals and settings relevant to their question? How much have they drawn on and collected evidence in terms of interviews, records, field notes, that are in principle capable of independent inspection by others? How much have they drawn on, whenever available or appropriate, quantitative evidence to check or test qualitative statements? To what extent do investigators seem to have sought out observations that might contradict or modify their analyses?[26, 29] It remains a matter of judgement for audiences of qualitative studies to determine how systematically investigators have approached such questions in assembling and interpreting their evidence. It is essential that qualitative researchers make more explicit the methods whereby their analyses have emerged so that audiences can make informed judgements about plausibility.

Understanding issues of quality of care

What is the role of qualitative research in understanding issues of quality of care? On the one hand, qualitative methods have enormous potential to illuminate how health care currently operates and the impact of care on patients. Thus puzzling issues such as the persistence of variations in clinical practice should be addressed by qualitative methods. How patients experience and benefit from health services also need examination by such methods. On the other hand, as more systematic evidence accumulates of effective interventions and appropriate forms of health care, another kind of application of qualitative methods is required. The changes in health services needed to promote quality are organisational and cultural and involve differing perspectives of a diverse range of health professionals, managers, and patients. Mechanisms of change such as clinical audit, quality assurance, and the adoption of clinical guidelines are social processes with meanings to participants that we need to understand. In such a complex environment qualitative methodology will be essential to give us models of how organisations change and innovate to adopt quality in health care.

There is an exciting range of qualitative methods capable of providing basic understanding of the processes and outcomes of health care. Rigorous and transparent attention to methodology is needed to convince audiences of the value of insights into the "black box" of health care. An understanding of these methods will in turn promote a fuller appreciation of the insights they can provide.

References

1. Pryce-Jones M. Critical incident technique as a method of assessing patient satisfaction. In: Fitzpatrick R, Hopkins A, eds. *Measurement of patients' satisfaction with their care*. London: Royal College of Physicians of London, 1993:87–98.
2. Fitzpatrick R, Hopkins A. Illness behaviour and headache, and the sociology of consultations for headache. In: Hopkins A, ed. *Headache: problems in management*. London: 1988:351–85.
3. Fitzpatrick R, Hopkins A. Patient satisfaction in relation to clinical care: a neglected contribution. In: Fitzpatrick R, Hopkins A, eds. *Measurement of patients' satisfaction with their care*. London: Royal College of Physicians of London, 1993:77–86.
4. Anderson R, Bury, M, eds. *Living with chronic illness*. London: Unwin Hyman, 1988.
5. Black N, Thompson E. Obstacles to medical audit: British doctors speak. *Soc Sci Med* 1993;**36**:849–56.
6. Daly J. Innocent murmurs: echocardiography and the diagnosis of cardiac normality. *Sociology of Health and Illness* 1989;**11**:99–116.
7. Green J. The views of singlehanded general practitioners: a qualitative study. BMJ 1993;**307**:607–10.
8. Morgan D, Krueger R. When to use focus groups and why. In: Morgan D, ed. *Successful focus groups*. London: Sage, 1993:3–19.
9. Morgan D. Future directions for focus groups. In: Morgan D, ed. *Successdful focus groups*. London: Sage, 1993:225–44.
10. de Vries H, Weijts W, Dijkstra M, Kok G. The utilisation of qualitative and quantitative data for health education program planning, implementation and evaluation, a spiral approach. *Health Educ Q* 1992;**19**:101–15.
11. NHS Management Executive. *Local voices*. London: Department of Health, 1992.

12 Murray S, Tapson J, Tumbull L, McCallum J, Little A. Listening to local voices: adapting rapid appraisal to assess health and social needs in general practice. *BMJ* 1994;**308**:698–700.

13 Van de Ven A, Delbecq A. The nominal group technique as a research instrument for exploratory health studies. *Am J Public Health* 1972;**62**:337–42.

14 Hunter D, McKee C, Sanderson C, Black N. Appropriate indications for prostatectomy in the UK – results of a consensus panel. J *Epidemiol Community Health* 1994;**48**:58–64.

15 Scott E, Black N. When does consensus exist in expert panels?*J Public Health* 1991;**13**:35–9.

16 Goffman E. *Asylums: essays on the social situation of mental patients and other inmates.* New York: Anchor, 1961.

17 Strong P. *The ceremonial order of the clinic.* London: Routledge, 1979.

18 Packwood T, Keen J, Buxton M. *Hospitals in transition: the resource management experiment.* Milton Keynes: Open University Press, 1991.

19 Pollitt C, Harrison S, Hunter D, Marnoch G. General management in the NHS: the initial impact, 1983-88. *Public Administration* 1991;**69**:61–83.

20 Bloor M. On the analysis of observational data: a discussion of the worth and use of inductive techniques and respondent validation. *Sociology* 1978;**12**:545–52.

21 Fielding N, Lee R, eds. *Using computers in qualitative research.* London: Sage, 1991.

22 Humphrey C, Berrow D. Developing role of medical audit advisory groups. *Quality in Health Care* 1993;**2**:232–38.

23 Pound P, Bury M, Gompertz P, Ebrahim S. Views of survivors of stroke on the benefits of physiotherapy. *Quality in Health Care* 1994;**3**:69–74.

24 Bryman A, Burgess R. Developments in qualitative data analysis: an introduction. In: Bryman A, Burgess R, eds. *Analysing qualitative data.* London: Routledge, 1993:1–15.

25 Crabtree B, Miller W, eds. *Doing qualitative research: multiple strategies.* London: Sage, 1993.

26 Silverman D. *Interpreting qualitative data.* London: Sage, 1993.

27 Bryman A, Burgess R, eds. *Analysing qualitative data.* London: Routledge, 1993.

28 Strauss A. *Qualitative analysis for social scientists.* Cambridge: Cambridge University Press, 1987.

29 Dingwall R. "Don't mind him – he's from Barcelona:" qualitative methods in health studies. In: Daly J, McDonald I, Willis B, eds.*Researching health care.* London: Routledge, 1992:161–75.

ARTICLE 10

THEORY AND METHOD IN QUALITATIVE RESEARCH

Beginning Research

Silverman, D

Chapter 1, Interpreting Qualitative Data: Methods for Analysing Talk, Text and Interaction, London: Sage, 1993

This is a text on qualitative methodology. However, any methodology only makes sense if we understand what the research process is all about. We will, therefore, begin this chapter by exploring the nature of social research.

In doing so, we will consider the following two issues:

1 How to generate a research problem.
2 The variety of qualitative methods.

At the outset, it helps to clarify our terms. In this chapter, we shall be discussing theories, hypotheses, methods and methodologies. In Table 1.1, I set out how each term will be used.

As we see from Table 1.1, theories provide a set of explanatory concepts. These concepts offer ways of looking at the world which are essential in defining a research problem. As we shall see shortly, without a theory, there is nothing to research. In social research, examples of such theories are *functionalism* (which looks at the functions of social institutions), *behaviourism* (which defines all behaviour in terms of 'stimulus' and 'response') and *symbolic interactionism* (which focusses on how we attach symbolic meanings to interpersonal relations).

So theories provide the impetus for research. As living entities, they are also developed and modified by good research. However, as used here, theories are never disproved but only found more or less useful.

This last feature distinguishes theories from hypotheses. Unlike theories, hypotheses are tested in research. Examples of hypotheses, considered later in this book, are:

• that how we receive advice is linked to how advice is given

• that responses to an illegal drug depend upon what one learns from others
• that voting in union elections is related to non-work links between union members.

As we shall see, a feature of many qualitative research studies is that there is no specific hypothesis at the outset but that hypotheses are produced (or induced) during the early stages of research. In any event, unlike theories, hypotheses can, and should, be tested. Therefore, we assess a hypothesis by its validity or truth.

A methodology is a general approach to studying a research topic. It establishes how one will go about studying any phenomenon. In social research, examples of methodologies are *positivism* (which seeks to discover laws using quantitative methods) and, of course, *qualitative methodology* (which is often concerned with inducing hypotheses from field research). Like theories, methodologies cannot be true or false, only more or less useful.

Finally, methods are specific research techniques. These include quantitative techniques, like statistical correlations, as well as techniques like observation, interviewing and audio-recording. Once again, in themselves, techniques are not true or false. They are more or less useful, depending on their fit with the theories and methodologies being used, the hypothesis being tested and/or the research topic that is selected. So, for instance, positivists will favour quantitative methods and interactionists often prefer to gather their data by observation. But, depending upon the hypothesis being tested, positivists may sometimes use qualitative methods – for instance in the exploratory

Table 1.1:

Basic Concepts in Research

Concept	Meaning	Relevance
Theory	A set of explanatory concepts	Usefulness
Hypothesis	A testable proposition	Validity
Methodology	A general approach to studying research topics	Usefulness
Method	A specific research technique	Good fit with theory, hypothesis and methodology

ARTICLE 11

stage of research. Equally, interactionists may sometimes use simple quantitative methods, particularly when they want to find an overall pattern in their data.

Having set out some basic concepts, we can now turn to the first issue to be discussed in this chapter.

USING THEORY TO GENERATE A RESEARCH PROBLEM

After long experience in supervising research, at both undergraduate and graduate levels, I find that beginning researchers tend to make two basic errors. First, they fail to distinguish sufficiently between research problems and problems that are discussed in the world around us. The latter kind of problems, which I shall call 'social problems', are at the heart of political debates and fill the more serious newspapers. However, although social problems, like unemployment, homelessness and racism, are important, by themselves they cannot provide a researchable topic.

The second error to which I have referred is sometimes related to the first. It arises where apprentice researchers take on an impossibly large research problem. For instance, it is important to find the causes of a social problem like homelessness, but such a problem is beyond the scope of a single researcher with limited time and resources. Moreover, by defining the problem so widely, one is usually unable to say anything in great depth about it.

As I tell my students, your aim should be to say 'a lot about a little (problem)'. This means avoiding the temptation to say 'a little about a lot'. Indeed, the latter path can be something of a 'cop-out'. Precisely because the topic is so wide-ranging, one can flit from one aspect to another without being forced to refine and test each piece of analysis.

In this part of the chapter, I shall focus on the first of these errors – the tendency to choose social problems as research topics. However, in recommending solutions to this error, I shall imply how one can narrow down a research topic.

What Is a Problem?

One has only to open a newspaper or to watch the television news to be confronted by a host of social problems. As I write, the British news media are full of references to a 'wave' of crimes committed by children – from the theft of cars to the murder of old people and other children. There are also several stories about how doctors infected by HIV have continued to work and, by implication, have endangered their patients.

The stories have this in common: both assume some sort of moral decline in which families or schools fail to discipline children and in which physicians fail to take seriously their professional responsibilities. In turn, the way each story is told implies a solution: tightening up 'discipline' in order to combat the 'moral decline'. However, before we can consider such a 'cure', we need to consider carefully the 'diagnosis'. Has juvenile crime increased or is the apparent increase a reflection of what

counts as a 'good' story? Alternatively, might the increase be an artifact of what crimes get reported? Again, how many health care professionals have actually infected their patients with HIV? I know of only one (disputed) case – a Florida dentist. Conversely, there is considerable evidence of patients infecting the medical staff who treat them. Moreover, why focus on HIV when other conditions like hepatitis B are far more infectious? Could it be that we hear so much about HIV because it is associated with 'stigmatised' groups?

However, apparent 'social' problems are not the only problems that may clamour for the attention of the researcher. Administrators and managers point to 'problems' in their organisations and may turn to social scientists for solutions.

It is tempting to allow such people to define a research problem particularly as there is usually a fat research grant attached to it! However, we must first look at the terms which are being used to define the problem. For instance, many managers will define problems in their organisation as problems of 'communication'. The role of the researcher is then to work out how people can communicate 'better'.

Unfortunately, talking about 'communication problems' raises many difficulties. For instance, it may deflect attention from the communication 'skills' inevitably used in interaction. It may also tend to assume that the solution to any problem is more careful listening, while ignoring power relations present inside and outside patterns of communication. Such relations may also make the characterisation of 'organisational efficiency' very problematic. Thus 'administrative' problems give no more secure basis for social research than do 'social' problems.

Of course, this is not to deny that there are any real problems in society. However, even if we agree about what these problems are, it is not clear that they provide a researchable topic, particularly for the apprentice researcher.

Take the case of the problems of people infected with HIV. Some of these problems are, quite rightly, brought to the attention of the public by the organised activities of groups of people who carry the infection. What social researchers can contribute are the particular theoretical and methodological skills of their discipline. So economists can research how limited health care resources can be used most effectively in coping with the epidemic in the West and in the Third World. Among sociologists, survey researchers can investigate patterns of sexual behaviour in order to try to promote effective health education, while qualitative methods may be used to study what is involved in the 'negotiation' of safer sex or in counselling people about HIV and AIDS.

The Trap of Absolutism

At last, by showing what social research *can* do, we seem to be hitting a positive note. However, there is one further trap which lies in our path when we are trying to define a research problem. What I call the 'absolutist' trap arises in the temptation to accept uncritically the conventional wisdoms of our day. Let me list the four such 'wisdoms' I will be considering:

- 'scientism'
- 'progress'
- 'tourism'
- 'romanticism'.

The first two issues mainly relate to quantitative social scientists; the last two are more of a problem for qualitative researchers.

Scientism: This involves uncritically accepting that 'science' is both highly distinct from, and superior to, 'common sense'. For instance, the quantitative researcher might study the relationship between the 'efficiency' of an organisation and its management 'structure'. The aim might be to get a more reliable and valid picture than we might get from 'common sense'.

However, what is 'efficient' and what is the management 'structure' cannot be separated from what the participants in the organisation do themselves. So, 'efficiency' and 'structure' are not stable realities but are defined and redefined in different organisational contexts (e.g. internal meetings, labour-management negotiations, press releases, etc.). Moreover, the researchers themselves will, inevitably, use their common-sense knowledge of how organisations operate in order to define and measure these 'variables' (see Cicourel: 1968, Silverman: 1975a).

This is *not* to say that there is no difference between 'science' and 'common sense'. Of course, social science needs to study how 'common sense' works in a way which 'common sense' would not and could not follow for itself. In doing so, however, it will inevitably draw upon common-sense knowledge. Scientism's mistake is to position itself entirely apart from, and superior to, 'common sense'.

Progress: In the nineteenth century, scientists believed they could detect a path leading towards 'progress' in history (e.g. Darwin on 'the origin of species', Marx on the inevitability of the demise of 'regressive' economic systems). This belief was maintained, with some modifications after the experiences of the two world wars, well into the twentieth century.

However, an uncritical belief in 'progress' is an unacceptable basis for scientific research. For instance, it is dangerous to assume that we can identify social progress when doctors listen more to their patients (Silverman: 1987, Ch. 8), when prison inmates are offered parole or when all of us feel freer to discuss our sexuality (Foucault: 1977, 1979). In each case, if we assume 'progress', then we may fail to identify the 'double-binds' of any method of communication and/or new forms of power.

Both 'scientism' and a commitment to 'progress' have had most impact on quantitative researchers. I now turn to two traps that have had a more direct influence on qualitative research.

Tourism: I have in mind the 'up-market' tourist who travels the world in search of encounters with alien cultures. Disdaining package tours and even the label of 'tourist', such a person has an insatiable thirst for the 'new' and 'different'.

The problem is that there are worrying parallels between the qualitative researcher and this kind of tourist. Such researchers often begin without a hypothesis and, like the tourist, gaze rapaciously at social scenes for signs of activities that appear to be new and different.

The danger in all this is that 'touristic' researchers may so focus on cultural and 'sub-cultural' (or group) differences that they fail to recognise similarities between the culture to which they belong and the cultures which they study. As Moernian (1974) noted in his study of a tribe in Thailand, once you switch away from asking 'leading' questions (which assume cultural differences) to observation of what people actually are doing, then you may find certain *common* features between social patterns in the West and East (see Chapter 9, pp. 196–197).

Romanticism: Just as the nineteenth century was the age of 'progress', so it was the time in which people expected that literature, art and music would express the inner world of the artist and engage the emotions of the audience. This movement was called 'romanticism'. As I later argue, there is a hint of this romanticism in some contemporary qualitative research (Chapter 9, pp. 197-210). This particularly applies where the researcher sets out to record faithfully the 'experiences' of some, usually disadvantaged, group (e.g. battered women, gay men, the unemployed, etc.).

As I later suggest, the romantic approach is appealing but dangerous. It may neglect how 'experience' is shaped by cultural forms of representation. For instance, what we think is most personal to us ('guilt', 'responsibility') may be simply a culturally given way of understanding the world (see my discussion of the mother of a young diabetic person in Chapter 6, pp. 121-122). So it is problematic to justify research in terms of its 'authentic' representation of 'experience' when what is 'authentic' is culturally defined,

This argument has implications for analysing interview data which I touch upon below. For the moment, I will conclude this section on generating a research problem by examining how different kinds of sensitivity can provide a solution to the twin traps of 'absolutism' and sliding into societal versions of 'social problems'.

Sensitivity and Researchable Problems

The various perspectives of social science provide a sensitivity to many issues neglected by those who define 'social' or administrative 'problems'. At the same time, it is possible to define and study any given research topic without falling into the 'absolutist' trap.

Let me distinguish four types of sensitivity:

- historical
- cultural
- political
- contextual.

I will explain and discuss each of these in turn.

Historical sensitivity: I have already implied how we can use this kind of sensitivity by looking critically at assumptions of 'progress' in society This means that, wherever possible, we should examine the relevant historical evidence when we are setting up a topic to research. For instance, in the 1950s and 1960s it was assumed that the 'nuclear family' (parents and children) had replaced the 'extended family' (many generations living together in the same household) of pre-industrial societies. Researchers simply seemed to have forgotten that lower life-expectancy may have made the 'extended family' pattern relatively rare in the past.

Again, historical sensitivity helps us to understand how we are governed. For instance, until the eighteenth century, the majority of the population were treated as a threatening 'mob' to be controlled, where necessary, by the use of force. Today, we are seen as individuals with 'needs' and 'rights' which must be understood and protected by society (see Foucault: 1977). But, although oppressive force may be used only rarely, we may be controlled in more subtle ways. Think of the knowledge about each of us contained in computerised data-banks and the pervasive video-cameras which record movements in many city streets. Historical sensitivity thus offers us multiple research topics which evade the 'absolutist' trap.

Cultual sensitivity: This form of sensitivity is a healthy antidote to the 'romantic' impulse. The latter impulse directs our attention to the unique experiences of individuals. Cultural sensitivity reveals how such experiences are shaped by given forms of representation.

For instance, in a study to which I shall return in greater detail (Chapter 4, pp. 73-75), Propp (1968) shows how all narratives may have a common structure deriving from the fairy story. Equally, Baruch (1982) reveals how mothers of handicapped children tell stories which appeal to their 'responsibility' in the face of adversity (Chapter 5, pp. 108114). In both cases, we are provided with a way of turning our studies of texts or interviews into highly researchable topics.

Political sensitivity: Allowing the current media 'scares' to determine our research topics is just as fallible as designing research in accordance with administrative or managerial interests. In neither case do we use political sensitivity to detect the vested interests behind this way of formulating a problem. The media, after all, need to attract an audience. Administrators need to be seen to be working efficiently.

So political sensitivity seeks to grasp the politics behind defining topics in particular ways. In turn, it helps in suggesting that we research how 'social problems' arise. For instance, Barbara Nelson (1984) looked at how 'child abuse' became defined as a recognisable problem in the late 1960s. She shows how the findings of a doctor about 'the battered baby syndrome' were adopted by the conservative Nixon administration through linking social problems to parental 'maladjustment' rather than to the failures of social programmes.

Political sensitivity does not mean that social scientists argue that there are no 'real' problems in society. Instead, it suggests that social science can make an important contribution to society by querying how 'official' definitions of problems arise. To be truthful, however, we should also recognise how social scientists often need to accept tacitly such definitions in order to attract research grants.

Contextual sensitivity: This is the least selfexplanatory and most contentious category in the present list. By 'contextual' sensitivity, I mean two things: (a) the recognition that apparently uniform institutions like 'the family', 'a tribe' or 'science' take on a variety of meanings in different contexts; (b) the understanding that participants in social life actively produce a context for what they do and that social researchers should not simply import their own assumptions about what context is relevant in any situation.

Point (a) above is reflected most obviously in Gubrium's (1992) work on the family and Gilbert and Mulkay's (1983) study of scientists (see Chapter 3 pp. 5658, and Chapter 9, pp. 200202). In both cases, fruitful research topics are suggested in regard to how apparently unitary institutions assume a variable meaning according to the participants' practical purposes (e.g. social workers or lawyers discussing 'family life'; scientists discussing science in published papers or in casual conversation).

Point (b) implies that we must carefully inspect what people do and say to see how, if at all, participants organise their activities in terms of particular categories or institutions (see Schegloff: 1991). Once again, it is highly suggestive in generating possible research topics. For instance, it suggests that we reformulate questions about the *impact* of context on behaviour into questions about how participants actively produce contexts for what they are doing together.

Both points are contentious because so much social science, like common sense, takes for granted the existence of stable institutions ('the family') and identities (gender, ethnicity etc.). This is most clearly seen in quantitative studies which correlate identity-based variables (e.g. the relationship between gender and occupation). However, it is also present in qualitative studies that demand that we interpret their observations in terms of assumed social contexts.

One final point in this section. The four kinds of sensitivity we have been considering offer different, sometimes contradictory, ways of generating research topics. I am not suggesting that all should be used at the beginning of any research study. However, if we are not sensitive to *any* of these issues, then we run the danger of lapsing into a 'social-problem'-based way of defining our research topics.

The Variety of Qualitative Methods

There are four major methods used by qualitative researchers:

Observation
Analysing texts and documents
Interviews
Recording and transcribing.

These methods are often combined. For instance, many case-studies combine observation with interviewing. Moreover, each method can be used in either qualitative or quantitative research studies. As Table 1.2 shows, the overall nature of the research methodology shapes how each method is used.

Table 1.2 underlines the point made in Table 1.1: methods are techniques which take on a specific meaning according to the methodology in which they are used.

So, in quantitative research, observation is not generally seen as a very important method of data collection. This is because it is difficult to conduct observational studies on large samples. Quantitative researchers also argue that observation is not a very 'reliable' data-collection method because different observers may record different observations. If used at all, observation is held to be only appropriate at a preliminary or 'exploratory' stage of research.

Conversely, observational studies have been fundamental to much qualitative research. Beginning with the pioneering case-studies of non Western societies by early anthropologists (Malinowski: 1922, Radcliffe-Brown: 1948) and continuing with the work by sociologists in Chicago prior to the Second World War (Thomas and Znaniecki: 1927), the observational method has often been the chosen method to understand another culture.

These contrasts are also apparent in the treatment of texts and documents. Quantitative researchers try to analyse written material in a way which will produce reliable evidence about a large sample. Their favoured method is 'content analysis' in which the researchers establish a set of categories and then count the number of instances that fall into each category. The crucial requirement is that the categories are sufficiently precise to enable different coders to arrive at the same results when the same body of material (e.g. newspaper headlines) are examined (see Berelson: 1952).

In qualitative research, small numbers of texts and documents may be analysed for a very different purpose. The aim is to understand the participants' categories and to see how these are used in concrete activities like telling stories (Propp: 1968, Sacks: 1974), assembling files (Cicourel: 1968, Gubrium and Buckholdt: 1982) or describing 'family life' (Gubrium: 1992). The reliability of the analysis is less frequently addressed. Instead, qualitative researchers make claims about their ability to reveal the local practices through which given 'end-products' (stories, files, descriptions) are assembled.

Interviews are commonly used in both methodologies. Quantitative researchers administer interviews or questionnaires to random samples of the population; this is referred to as 'survey research'. 'Fixed-choice' questions (e.g. 'yes' or 'no') are usually preferred because the answers they produce lend themselves to simple tabulation, unlike 'open-ended' questions which produce answers which need to be subsequently coded. A central methodological issue for quantitative researchers is the reliability of the interview schedule and the representativeness of the sample.

For instance, after surveys of voting intention did not coincide with the result of the British General Election of 1992, survey researchers looked again at their methodology. Assuming that some respondents in the past may have lied to interviewers about their voting intentions, some companies now provide a ballot box into which respondents put mock ballot slips thereby eliminating the need to reveal one's preferences to the interviewer. Attention is also being given to assembling

Table 1.2:

Different Uses for Four Methods

Method	Methodology	
	Quantitative research	Qualitative research
Observation	Preliminary work, e.g. prior to framing questionnaire	Fundamental to understanding another culture
Textual analysis	Content analysis, i.e. counting in terms of researchers' categories	Understanding participants' categories
Interviews	'Survey research': mainly fixed-choice questions to random samples	'Open-ended' questions to small samples
Transcripts	Used infrequently to check the accuracy of interview records	Used to understand how participants organise their talk

a more representative sample to interview, bearing in mind the expense of a completely random sample of the whole British population.

'Authenticity' rather than reliability is often the issue in qualitative research. The aim is usually to gather an 'authentic' understanding of people's experiences and it is believed that 'open-ended' questions are the most effective route towards this end. So, for instance, in gathering life histories or in interviewing parents of handicapped children (Baruch: 1982), people may simply be asked: 'tell me your story'. Qualitative interview studies are often conducted with small samples and the interviewer-interviewee relationship may be defined in political rather than scientific terms (e.g Finch: 1984).

Finally, transcripts of audio-recordings are rarely used in quantitative research, probably because of the assumption that they are difficult to quantify. Conversely, as we shall see (Chapter 6), audio-recordings are an increasingly important part of qualitative research. Transcripts of such recordings, based on standardised conventions, provide an excellent record of 'naturally occurring' interaction. Compared to fieldnotes of observational data, recordings and transcripts can offer a highly reliable record to which researchers can return as they develop new hypotheses.

This rather abstract presentation can now be made more concrete by examining a number of qualitative studies using each method. I will take the example of research on social aspects of AIDS because it is a highly discussed, contemporary topic and an area in which I have worked. For each study presented, I will show how different theoretical and methodological imperatives shaped the choice and use of the method concerned.

Observation

In 1987, I began sitting in at a weekly clinic held at the Genito-Urinary Department of an English inner-city hospital (Silverman: 1989c). The clinic's purpose was to monitor the progress of HIV-positive patients who were taking the drug AZT (Retrovir). AZT then seemed able to slow down the rate at which the virus reproduces itself.

Like any observational study, the aim was to gather first-hand information about social processes in a 'naturally occurring' context. No attempt was made to interview the individuals concerned because the focus was upon what they actually did in the clinic rather than upon what they thought about what they did. The researcher was present in the consulting-room at a side-angle to both doctors and patient.

Patients' consent for the researcher's presence was obtained by the senior doctor. Given the presumed sensitivity of the occasion, tape-recording was not attempted. Instead, detailed handwritten notes were kept, using a separate sheet for each consultation.

The sample was small (fifteen male patients seen in thirty-seven consultations over seven clinic sessions) and no claims were made about its representativeness. Because observational methods were rare in this area, the study was essentially exploratory. However, as we

shall see, an attempt was made to link the findings to other social research about doctor-patient relations.

As Sontag (1979) has noted, illness is often taken as a moral or psychological metaphor. The major finding of the study was the moral baggage attached to being HIV-positive. For instance, many patients used a buzzer to remind them to take their medication during the night. As one commented (P = Patient):

P: It's a dead giveaway. Everybody knows what you've got.

However, despite the social climate in which HIV infection is viewed, there was considerable variation in how people presented themselves to the medical team. Four styles of 'self-presentation' (Goffman: 1959) were identified. Each style is briefly noted below:

'Cool': Here even worrying medical statements were treated with an air of politeness and acceptance rather than concern or apparent anxiety. For example, one patient generally answered all questions in monosyllables.

His only sustained intervention was when he asked about the name of a doctor he would be seeing at another hospital for his skin infection. He made no comment when a doctor observed that AZT was keeping him alive.

'Anxiety': At the other extreme, some patients treated even apparent greetings as an oppotunity to display 'anxiety'. For instance:

Dr: How are you?
P: Heh. Pretty weak. Something I can't put my finger on. Not right. Don't know.

'Objective'; As has been noted in other studies (see Baruch: 1982, discussed in Chapter 5, pp. 108-114), health professionals commonly present themselves to doctors as bundles of objective symptoms. One such professional, who was a patient in this clinic, behaved in exactly this way. For instance:

P: I was wondering whether Acyclovir in connection with the AZT might cause neutropenia . . . (describing his herpes symptoms). It was interesting. So you'd suggest it four times a day. Because normally they recommend five times a day.

'Theatrical': One way of responding to questions about one's physical condition was to downplay them in order to make observations about social situations, acknowledging the listening audience. For instance:

Dr: How are you feeling physically?
P: Fine. The other thing was. . . (account of doctor who didn't wave to him in the street). He's just a bloody quack like you. No offence.
[to researcher and medical student]
I'm a bad case by the way so don't take no notice of me

Three important points need to be made about this discussion. First, there was no simple correspondence between each patient and a particular 'style' of self-presentation. Rather, each way of presenting oneself was available to each patient within any one consultation, where it might have a particular social function. So the focus was on social processes rather than on psychological states. Second, I have only been to able to offer brief extracts to support my argument. As we shall see in Chapter 7, such use of evidence has led to doubts about the validity or accuracy of qualitative research.

My third point is that these findings reflect only part of the study. We also discovered how the ethos of 'positive thinking' was central to many patients' accounts and how doctors systematically concentrated on the 'bodies' rather than the 'minds' of their patients – we get a sense of this in the extract immediately above where the patient resists an attempt by the doctor to get him to talk more about his physical condition. This led on to some practical questions about the division of labour between doctors and counsellors.

Textual Analysis

Kitzinger and Miller (1992) have looked at the relation between media reporting of AIDS and the audience's understanding. Their analysis of British television news bulletins provides a good example of how textual analysis may be used in qualitative research on social aspects of AIDS. It also shows how qualitative researchers try to avoid questions deriving from 'social problem' perspectives, while recognising that phenomena are always socially defined. Kitzinger and Miller's concern with the social definition of phenomena is shown by the inverted commas they place around concepts like 'AIDS', 'Africa' and what is 'really' the case. As the authors explain:

> This chapter focusses on audiences and the role of the media in changing, reinforcing or contributing to ideas about AIDS, Africa and race. It does not argue that HIV either does or not originate in Africa . . . Here we are not directly addressing questions about where the virus 'really' came from or the actual distribution of infection. Instead we are focussing on how different *answers* to these questions are produced, framed and sustained, what these tell us about the construction of 'AIDS' and 'Africa' and what socio-political consequences they carry with them. (Kitzinger and Miller: 1992, 28, my emphasis)

Over three years of television news reports were examined. In one such report, statistics on HIV infection were given for the whole of Africa and a map of Africa was shown with the word 'AIDS' fixed across the continent. The map was also stamped with the words '3 Million Sufferers'.

In the three-year period, the only country to be distinguished as different from the rest of Africa was South Africa. Indeed, on one occasion, South Africa was

described as 'holding the line' against an HIV invasion from black Africa. By contrast, images of black Africans with AIDS were used in all the news reports studied. Moreover, the spread of the epidemic was related to 'traditional sexual values' or, more generally, to 'African culture'.

To see how these media images impacted upon their audience, many discussion groups were established among people with particular occupations (e.g. nurses, police, teachers), perceived 'high involvement' in the issue (e.g. gay men, prisoners) and 'low involvement' (e.g. retired people, students).

Although members of all groups were sceptical about media coverage of news issues, they nonetheless accepted the general assumption that AIDS came from Africa and is prevalent there. White people usually began from the assumption that Africa is a hotbed of sexually transmitted diseases. This was based on the belief that sexual intercourse typically begins at an early age and that sexual diseases are spread through polygamy.

However, not all individuals shared these beliefs. Kitzinger and Miller refer to several factors which led people to doubt the media treatment. Among these were the following: personal contact with alternative information from trusted individuals or organisations, personal experience of being 'scapegoated', personal experience of conditions in Africa and being black yourself. The authors conclude:

> Our research shows both the power of the media and the pervasiveness of stock white cultural images of black Africa; it is easy to believe that Africa is a reservoir of HIV infection because 'it fits'. Journalists draw on these cultural assumptions when they produce reports on AIDS and Africa. But, in so doing, they are helping to reproduce and legitimise them. (*ibid*, 49)

Kitzinger and Miller's study has a much bigger data-base than my study of one medical clinic. However, it shares two features in common. First, in both studies, the researchers began without a hypothesis. Instead, as in much qualitative research, they sought to induce and then test hypotheses during their data-analyses. Second, both studies were theoretically driven by the assumption that social phenomena derive their meaning from how they are defined by participants. Both these features are found in the remaining two studies we shall consider.

Interviews

Weatherburn *et al* (1992) note that many studies assert that there is an association between alcohol and drug 'misuse' and 'risky' sexual behaviour. Conversely, Weatherburn *et al* suggest the following: 'the link is asserted but not proven; that the evidence is at best contradictory and that this assertion is informed by a puritanical moral agenda' (119).

In their own research, we find two assumptions which are absent from these earlier, generally (quantitative, research studies:

1 No assumption is made about a strong interrelation between alcohol use and engagement in unsafe sex.
2 Psychological traits (like defects of character or weakness of resolve under the influence of alcohol) are held to be an inadequate explanation of enduring unsafe sexual practices (*ibid*, 122–123).

Weatherburn *et al*'s research is part of Project SIGMA which is a British longitudinal study of a non-clinic-based cohort of over one thousand gay men. Like other qualitative researchers, they distrusted explanations of behaviour which reduced social life to a response to particular 'stimuli' or 'variables'. Consequently, they favoured 'open-ended' questions to try to understand the meanings attached to alcohol use by their sample. For instance:

> The first question asked respondents: 'Would you say alcohol plays a significant role in your sex life?' Those respondents who said 'yes' were probed in detail about its exact nature. Respondents were also asked whether alcohol had ever influenced them to engage in unsafe sexual behaviours. (*ibid*. 123)

Typically, in an open ended interview study, respondents were encouraged to offer their own definitions of particular activities, 'unsafe sex' for example.

The findings of the study reflect the complexity of the attempt to explain the 'causes' of social behaviour. The effects of alcohol were found to depend upon 'the context of the sexual encounter and the other party involved in the sexual negotiation' (129). Only in a minority of reports was alcohol treated as the 'cause' of unsafe behaviour. In the majority of cases, although people might report themselves as 'fairly drunk', they described their sexual activities as the outcome of conscious deliberation.

However, the authors raise a crucial issue about the meaning we should attach to such descriptions, given that people may recall those features that depict their behaviour as socially desirable: 'it is recognized that asking people retrospective questions about alcohol use may well be problematic, both because of social desirability phenomena and because alcohol itself impairs recall' (123).

As we shall see in Chapter 5, this observation goes to the heart of an unresolved debate about the status of interview accounts, namely are such accounts:

• true or false representations of such features as attitudes and behaviour?
• simply 'accounts', whose main interest lies in how they are constructed rather than their accuracy?

This interview study highlights the advantages of qualitative research in offering an apparently 'deeper' picture than the variable-based correlations of quantitative studies. However, it also implies why it can be difficult to get funding or acceptance for qualitative research. However questionable are the assumptions

behind some quantitative research, it tends to deliver apparently reliable and valid correlations between 'variables' that appear to be self-evident. Moreover, these correlations usually lead in clear-cut policy directions.

However, some qualitative research can combine sensitivity to participants' definitions with correlations carrying direct policy implications. We shall see this in our final research study.

Transcripts

Silverman *et al*'s (1992) study was based on audio-tapes of HIV/AIDS counselling from ten different medical centres in Britain, the U.S.A. and Trinidad. The focus was on advice (both how advice was given and how it was received). The interest in advice derived from three sources:

1 The research was part-funded by the English Health Education Authority: this meant that analysis of advice sequences would be appropriate to its interest in health promotion.
2 Early work on the project had identified two basic 'communication formats' through which such counselling was conducted; the analysis of 'information delivery' and interview formats provided a crucial resource for the analysis of how advice-giving worked (see Peräkylä and Silverman: 1991a).
3 A recent study by Heritage and Sefi (1992) of health visitors and mothers had provided important findings about the relationship between different forms of advice-giving and their uptake by the client.

As I show in Chapter 7 (p. 167), we were able to tabulate the relationship between the form in which advice was given and how it was received in fifty advice sequences. Broadly speaking, personalised advice, offered after clients had been asked to specify their concerns, was associated with a 'marked acknowledgment' (e.g. a comment on the advice or a further question from the client). Conversely, counsellors who gave generalised advice, without first getting their clients to specify a particular problem, generally received only 'unmarked acknowledgments' (e.g. 'mm', 'right', 'yes').

However, the availability of detailed transcripts meant that we could go beyond this predictable finding. In particular, we sought to address the functions of counsellors' behaviour – particularly given the fact that, if asked, many of them would have recognised that generalised advice giving is likely to be ineffective. We hoped, thereby, to make a constructive input into policy debates by examining the *functions* of communication sequences in a particular institutional context.

Let us look at a relevant data extract. The transcription symbols are provided in Chapter 6, p. 118:

ARTICLE 11

Extract 1.1

(C = Counsellor; P = Patient)

```
 1 C: .hhhh Now when someo:ne er is tested (.) and they
 2    ha:ve a negative test result .hh it's obviously
 3    idealuh:m that (.) they then look after themselves to
 4    prevent [any further risk of =
 5 P:        [Mm hm
 6 C: = infection. .hhhh I mean obviously this is only
 7    possible up to a point because if .hhh you get into
 8    a sort of serious relationship with someone that's
 9    long ter:m .hh you can't obviously continue to use
10    condoms forever. .hh Uh:m and a point has to come
11    where you make a sort of decision (.4) uh:m if you
12    are settling down about families and things that you
13    know (.6) you'd- not to continue safer sex.
14    [.hhhh Uh:m but obviously: (1.0) you =
15 P: [Mm:
16 C: =nee:d to be (.) uh:m (.) take precautions uhm (0.3)
17    and keep to the safer practices .hhh if: obviously
18    you want to prevent infection in the future.
```

```
19 P: [Mm hm
20 C: [.hhhh The problem at the moment is we've got it
21    here in [names City] in particular (.) right across
22    the boar:d you know from all walks of life.
23 P: Mm hm
24 C: Uh::m from you know (.) the sort of established high
25    r- risk groups (.) now we're getting heterosexual
26    (.) [transmission as well. .hh Uhm=
27 P:    [Mm hm
28 C: = so obviously everyone really needs to careful. .hhh
29    Now whe- when someone gets a positive test result
30    er: then obviously they're going to ke- think very
31    carefully about things. .hhhh Being MIV positive
32    doesn't necessarily mean that that person is going
33    to develop ai:ds (.) later on.
34    (.)
35 P: Mm hm
```

We can make three observations about this extract. First, C delivers advice without having elicited from P a perceived problem. Reasons of space do not allow us to include what immediately precedes this extract but it involves another topic (the meaning of a positive test result) and no attempt is made to question P about his possible response to this topic, i.e. how he might change his behaviour after a negative test result. Moreover, within this extract, C introduces fresh topics (what to do in a 'serious' relationship in lines 6-13; the spread of HIV in the city in lines 20–22) without attempting to elicit P's own perspectives.

Second, predictably, P only produces variations on 'mm hmm' in response to C's advice. While these may indicate that P is listening, they do not show P uptake and might be taken as a sign of passive resistance to the advice (see Heritage and Sefi: 1992).

Third, C does not personalise her advice. Instead of using a personal pronoun or the patient's name, she refers to 'someone' and 'they' (lines 1) and 'everyone' (line 28).

Advice sequences like these are very common at three out of the five counselling centres we have examined. So we have to ask ourselves why counsellors should use a format which is likely to generate so little patient uptake. Since our preference was not to criticise professionals but to understand the logic of their work, we need to look at the *functions* as well as the dysfunctions of this way of proceeding.

A part of the answer seems to lie in the content of the advice given. Note how in Extract 1.1 the counsellor is giving advice about what she tells patients *after* a particular test result. But the patient here does not yet have his result – indeed he has not yet even consented to the test. This leaves it open to the patient to treat what he is being told not as advice but as information delivery (about the advice C would give if P turned out to be seropositive or

seronegative). Moreover, throughout C avoids personalising her advice. Rather than saying what she advises P to do, she uses the non-specific term 'someone'.

All the available research suggest that behaviour change rarely occurs on the basis of information alone. Why, therefore, would counsellors want to package their advice in a way which makes patient uptake less likely?

A part of the answer to this question lies in the *dysfunctions* of recipient-designed advice. Throughout our corpus of interviews, counsellors exit quickly from *personalised* advice when patients offer only minimal responses like 'mm mm's. It seems that, if someone is giving you personalised advice, if you don't show more uptake than 'mm mm', this will be problematic to the advice-giver. Conversely, if you are merely giving somebody general information, then occasional 'mm mm's are all that is required for the speaker to continue in this format. Moreover, truncated, non-personalised advice sequences are also usually far shorter – an important consideration for hard-pressed counsellors.

Another function of offering advice in this way is that it neatly handles many of the issues of delicacy that can arise in discussing sexual behaviour. First, the counsellor can be heard as making reference to what she tells 'anyone' so that this particular patient need not feel singled out for attention about his private life. Second, because there is no step-by-step method of questioning, patients are not required to expand on their sexual practices with the kinds of hesitations we have found elsewhere in our research (Silverman and Peräkylä: 1990). Third, setting up advice sequences that can be heard as information delivery shields the counsellor from some of the interactional difficulties of appearing to tell strangers what they should be doing in the most intimate aspects of their behaviour. Finally, predictably, information-oriented counselling produces very little conflict. So in Extract 1.1, there is no active resistance from P. Indeed, topic follows topic with a remarkable degree of smoothness and at great speed.

So the character of HIV counselling as a focussed conversation on mostly delicate topics explains why truncated advice sequences (like that seen in Extract 1.1) predominate in our transcripts.

Clearly, such sequences are functional for *both* local and institutional contexts. This underlines the need to locate 'communication problems' in a broader structural context. Our research had much to say about how counsellors can organise their talk in order to maximise patient uptake. However, without organisational change, the impact of such communication techniques alone might be minimal or even harmful. For instance, encouraging patient uptake will usually involve longer counselling sessions. Experienced counsellors will tell you that, if they take so long with one client that the waiting period for others increases, some clients will simply walk out – and hence may continue their risky behaviour without learning their HIV-status.

Undoubtedly, then, there are gains for the counsellor in setting up advice-packages which are truncated and non-personalised. Obviously, however, there are concomitant losses of proceeding this way. As we have shown, such advice packages produce far less patient uptake and, therefore, their function in creating an environment in which people might re-examine their own sexual behaviour is distinctly problematic.

Two possible solutions suggest themselves from the data analysed by this study. First, avoiding necessarily 'delicate' and unstable advice sequences but encouraging patients to draw their own conclusions from a particular line of questioning. Second, since both this method and step-by-step advice-giving take considerable time, finding ways of making more time available for more effective counselling. I take up these matters in greater detail in Chapter 8

Having set out four different qualitative methods, I want to make two general observations. First, as I have emphasised, no research method stands on its own. So far, I have sought to show the link between methods and methodologies in social research. However, there is a broader, societal context in which methods are located and deployed. As a crude example, texts depended upon

the invention of the printing press or, in the case of television or audio-recordings, upon modern communication technologies.

Moreover, such activities as observation and interviewing are not unique to social researchers. For instance, as Foucault (1977) has noted, the observation of the prisoner has been at the heart of modern prison reform, while the method of questioning used in the interview reproduces many of the features of the Catholic confessional or the psycho-analytic consultation. Its pervasiveness is reflected by the centrality of the interview study in so much contemporary social research. In the two collections of papers from which the research studies above have been selected, for example, fourteen out of nineteen empirical studies are based on interview data. One possible reason for this may not derive from methodological considerations. Think, for instance, of how much interviews are a central (and popular) feature of mass media products, from 'talk shows' to 'celebrity' interviews. Perhaps, we all live in what might be called an 'interview society' in which interviews seem central to making sense of our lives.

All this means that we need to resist treating research methods as mere techniques. This is reflected in the attention paid in this book to the *analysis* of data rather than to methods of data-*collection*.

CONCLUSION

By focussing on the topics of HIV and AIDS, I have tried to show how four different research methods can be used in qualitative research. Despite the different kinds of data which they generate, they lead to a distinctive form of analysis which is centrally concerned with avoiding a 'social problem' perspective by asking how participants attach meaning to their activities and 'problems'.

Part Two of this book sets out each research method in greater detail and Part Three returns to issues of validity and relevance which are touched upon in this chapter. However, before we deal with these detailed issues, it will be helpful, in the light of the studies discussed here, to review what other writers have said about the distinctive properties of qualitative research. This is the topic of Chapter 2.

This chapter was first published by Sage Publications and is reproduced by permission of Sage Publications

DESIGNING QUALITATIVE STUDIES

Chapter 5, Qualitative evaluation and research methods, Newbury Park, Ca: Sage, 1990: 145-198

MQ Patton

The First Evaluation

The young people gathered around Halcolm. "Tell us again Teacher of Many Things, about the first evaluation."

"The first evaluation was conducted a long, long time ago," he began. It happened in Ancient Babylon when Nebuchadnezzar was King. Nebuchadnezzar had just conquered Jerusalem in the third year of the reign of Jehoiakim, King of Judah. Now Nebuchadnezzar was a shrewd ruler. He decided to bring carefully selected children of Israel into the palace for special training so that they might be more easily integrated into Chaldean culture. This special program was the forerunner, of the compensatory education programs that would become so popular in the twentieth century. The three year program was royally funded with special allocations and scholarships provided by Nebuchadnezzar. The ancient text from the Great Book records that

> the king spake unto Ashpenaz the master of his eunuchs that he should bring certain of the children of Israel, and of the King's seed, and of the princes; children in whom was no blemish, but well-favored and skillful in all wisdom, and cunning in knowledge, and understanding science, and such as had ability in them to stand in the king's palace, and whom they might teach the learning and the tongue of the Chaldeans.
>
> And the king appointed them a daily provision of the king's meat, and of the wine which he drank; so nourishing them three years, that at the end thereof they might stand before the king. (Daniel 1:3-5)

"Now this program had scarcely been established when the king found himself faced with a student rebellion led by a radical named Daniel, who decided for religious reasons that he would not consume the king's meat and wine. This created a real problem for the program administrator who was responsible to the king. If Daniel and his coconspirators did not eat their dormitory food, they might fare poorly in the program and endanger not only future program funding but also the program director's head! The Great Book says,

> But Daniel purposed in his heart that he would not defile himself with the portion of the king's meat, nor with the wine which he drank; therefore he requested of the prince of the eunuchs that he might not defile himself.
> And the prince of the eunuchs said unto Daniel, I

fear my lord the king, who hath appointed your meat and your drink; for why should he see your faces worse liking than the children which are of your sort? Then shall ye make me endanger my head to the king. (Daniel 1:8, 10)

"At this point, Daniel proposed history's first educational experiment and program evaluation. He and three friends would be placed on a strict vegetarian diet for ten days (nothing but "pulse" and water), while other students continued on the king's rich diet of meat and wine. At the end of ten days the program director would inspect the treatment group for any signs of physical deterioration and judge the productivity of Daniel's alternative diet plan. As Daniel described the experiment:

> Prove thy servants, I beseech thee, ten days; and let them give us pulse to eat, and water to drink. Then let our countenances be looked upon before thee, and the countenance of the children that eat the portion of the king's meat: and as thou seest, deal with thy servants. So he consented to them in this matter, and proved them ten days. (Daniel 1:12-14)

"During the ten days of waiting Ashpenaz had a terrible time. He couldn't sleep, he had no appetite, and he had trouble working because he was preoccupied worrying about how the evaluation would turn out. He had a lot at stake. Besides, in those days they hadn't quite worked out the proper division of labor so he had to play the roles of both program director and evaluator. You see . . ."

The young listeners interrupted Halcolm. They sensed that he was about to launch into a sermon on the origins of the division of labor when they still wanted to hear the end of the story about the origins of evaluation. "How did it turn out?" they asked. "Did Daniel end up looking, better or worse from the new diet? Did Ashpenaz lose his head?"

"Patience, patience," Halcolm pleaded. "Ashpenaz had no reason to worry The results were quite amazing. The Great Book says that

> at the end of ten days their countenances appeared fairer and fatter in flesh than all the children which did eat the portion of the king's meat.
>
> Thus Melzar took away the portion of their meat, and the wine that they should drink; and gave them pulse.

As for these four children, God gave them
knowledge and skill in all learning and wisdom;
and Daniel had understanding in all visions and
dreams. Now at the end of the days that the king
had said he should bring them in, then the prince
of the eunuchs brought them in before
Nebuchadnezzar. And in all matters of wisdom
and understanding, that the king inquired of
them, he found them ten times better than all the
magicians and astrologers that were in all his
realm. (Daniel 1:15–18, 20)

"And that, my children, is the story of the first
evaluation. Those were the good old days when
evaluations really got used. Made quite a difference to
Ashpenaz and Daniel. Now off with you – and see if you
can do as well."
– From *Halcolm's Evaluation Histories*

A Meta-Evaluation

A meta-evaluation is an evaluation of an evaluation. A
great deal can be learned about evaluation designs by
conducting a meta-evaluation of history's first program
evaluation. Let us imagine a panel of experts conducting
a rigorous critique of this evaluation of Babylon's
compensatory education program for Israeli students:

(1) small sample size (n = 4);
(2) selectivity bias because recruitment into the
    program was done by "creaming," that is, only the
    best prospects among, the Children of Israel were
    brought into the program;
(3) selectivity bias because students were self-selected
    into the treatment group (diet of pulse and water);
(4) failure to clearly specify and control the nature of
    the treatment, thus allowing for the possibility of
    treatment contamination – we don't know what
    other things aside from a change in diet either
    group was involved in that might have explained
    the outcomes observed;
(5) possibility of interaction effects between the diet
    and the students' belief system and/or relationship
    to God;
(6) outcome criteria vague – just what is
    "countenance"?
(7) measures of outcomes poorly operationalized and
    nonstandardized;
(8) single observer with deep personal involvement in
    the program introduces possibility of selective
    perception and bias in the observations;
(9) validity and reliability data are not reported for the
    instruments used to measure the final, summative
    outcome ("he found them ten times better than all
    the magicians and astrologers . . ."); and
(10) possible reactive effects from the students'
    knowledge that they were being evaluated.

Despite all of these threats to internal validity, not to
mention external validity, the information generated by
the evaluation appears to have been used to make a major
decision about the program. Indeed, it is difficult to find a
more exemplary model for the utilization of research in
making educational policy decisions than this "first
evaluation" conducted under the auspices of
Nebuchadnezzar so many years ago. Immediately
following determination of the evaluation results a policy
decision was made to allow Daniel and friends to maintain
their diet of pulse and water. The longitudinal indicators
collected over the three year period suggest that the
decision was appropriate; Daniel did place first in his class.
This case study is an exemplar of evaluation research
having an immediate, decisive, and lasting impact on an
educational program. Modern evaluation researchers,
flailing away in seemingly futile efforts to affect
contemporary governmental decisions, can be forgiven a
certain nostalgia for the "good old days" in Babylon when
evaluation research really made a difference.

But should the results have been used? Given the
apparent weakness of the evaluation design, was it
appropriate to make a major program decision on the
basis of data generated by such a weak research design?

I would argue that not only was utilization
exemplary in this case, but the research design was also
exemplary. The evaluation design was exemplary
because the study was set up in such a way as to provide
precisely the information needed by the program
director to make the decision he needed to make.
Certainly, it is a poor research design to study the
relationship between nutrition and educational
achievement. It is even a poor design to decide if *all*
students should be placed on a vegetarian diet. But
those were not the issues. The question that the
program director had to deal with was whether to place
four specific students on a special diet at their request.
The information he needed concerned the consequences
of that specific change and *only* that specific change. He
showed no interest in generalizing the results beyond
those four students, and he showed no interest in
convincing others that the measures he made were valid
and reliable. He was the only person who had to trust
the measures used, and so data collection was designed
in such a way as to maximize his belief in the
meaningfulness of the observations. If any bias existed
in his observations, given what he had at stake, the bias
would have operated against a demonstration of positive
outcomes rather than in favor of such outcomes.

While there are hints of whimsy in the suggestion that
this first evaluation was exemplary, I do not mean to be
completely facetious. I am serious in suggesting that the
Babylonian example is an exemplar of utilization-focused
evaluation. It contains and illustrates all the factors
modern evaluation researchers have verified as critical
from studies of utilization (Patton, 1986). The decision
maker who was to use information generated by the
evaluation was clearly identified and deeply involved in
every stage of the evaluation process. The evaluation
question was carefully focused on needed information
that could be used in the making of a specific decision.
The evaluation methods and design were appropriately

matched to the evaluation question. The results were understandable, credible, and relevant. Feedback was immediate and utilization was decisive. Few modern evaluations can meet the high standards for evaluation set by Ashpenaz and Daniel more than 3,000 years ago.

This chapter discusses some ways in which research designs can be appropriately matched to evaluation questions in an attempt to emulate the exemplary match between evaluation problem and research design achieved in the Babylonian evaluation. As with previous chapters, I shall emphasize the importance of being both strategic and practical in creating evaluation designs. Being strategic begins with being clear about the purpose of the intended research or evaluation.

CLARITY ABOUT PURPOSE: A TYPOLOGY

Purpose is the controlling force in research. Decisions about design, measurement, analysis, and reporting all flow from purpose. Therefore, the first step in a research process is getting clear about purpose. The centrality of purpose in making methods decisions is evident from examining alternative purposes:

(1) *basic research*, to contribute to fundamental knowledge and theory;
(2) *applied research*, to illuminate a societal concern;
(3) *summative evaluation* to determine program effectiveness;
(4) *formative evaluation* to improve a program; and
(5) *action research* to solve a specific problem.

Basic and applied researchers publish in scholarly journals, where their audience is other researchers who will judge their contributions using disciplinary standards of rigor, validity, and theoretical import. In contrast, evaluators and action researchers publish reports for specific stakeholders who will use the results to make decisions, improve programs, and solve problems.

Standards for judging quality vary among these five different types of research. Expectations and audiences are different. Reporting and dissemination approaches are different. Because of these differences, the researcher must be clear at the beginning about which purpose has priority No single study can serve all of these different purposes and audiences equally well. With clarity about purpose and primary audience, the researcher can go on to make specific design, data-gathering, and analysis decisions to meet the priority purpose and address the intended audience.

In the Babylonian example, the purpose was simply to find out what would happen to four participants' countenances on a vegetarian diet. Not *why* it happened, but what. The research was, therefore, appropriately simple in design and descriptive for the purpose of making a minor program adjustment. No contribution to general knowledge. No testing or development of theory. No generalizations. No scholarly publication. No elaborate report on methods. Just find out what would happen to inform a single decision and solve a problem. The participants in the program were involved

in the research; indeed, the idea of putting the diet to an empirical test originated with Daniel. In short, we have a very nice example of *action research*.

The king's examination of program participants at the end of three years was quite different. We might infer that the king was judging the overall value of the program. Did it accomplish his objectives? Should it be continued? Could the outcomes he observed be attributed to the program? This is the kind of research we have come to call a *summative evaluation* – summing up judgments about a program to make a major decision about its value, whether it should be continued, and whether the demonstrated model can or should be generalized to and replicated for other participants or in other places.

Now imagine that researchers from the University of Babylon wanted to study the diet as a manifestation of culture in order to develop a theory about the role of diet in transmitting culture. Their sample, their data collection, their questions, the duration of fieldwork, and their presentation of results would all be quite different from the action research undertaken by Ashpenaz and Daniel. The university study would have taken much longer and yet would not have helped Ashpenaz make his simple decision. On the other hand, the action research done in ten days to solve a program problem would have been scoffed at by the University of Babylon researchers. Different purposes. Different criteria for judging the research contribution. Different methods. Different audiences. Different kinds of research.

These are examples of how purpose can vary. In the next section, I shall present a more formal framework For distinguishing these five different research purposes.

As a preface to the next section, let me share with the reader the quandary I experienced in deciding where to place this next section on purpose. It could logically be the opening section of the book, given that clarity about purpose is fundamental to all other methods decisions. Some instructors may reasonably decide to assign this section to be read first. But I preferred to take the reader right into examples of qualitative data in Chapter 1. By delaying this discussion of purpose until the fifth chapter, I have adopted an inductive strategy that parallels the induction in qualitative inquiry. Previous chapters have presented the nature of qualitative inquiry, philosophical and theoretical foundations, and practical applications. In effect, the reader has been presented with a large array of options, alternatives, and variations. *How does one sort it all out to decide what to do in a specific study? The answer is to get clear about purpose.* The framework that follows is meant to facilitate achieving this necessary clarity about purpose while also illustrating how one can organize a mass of observations into some coherent typology – a major analytical tool of qualitative inquiry. The sections that follow examine each type of research: basic research, applied research, summative evaluation research, formative evaluation, and action research.

Basic Research

The purpose of basic research is knowledge for the sake of knowledge. Researchers engaged in basic research want to understand how the world operates. They are interested in investigating a phenome non in order to get at the nature of reality with regard to that phenomenon. The basic researcher's purpose is to understand and explain.

Basic researchers typically work within specific disciplines, such as physics, biology, psychology, economics, geography, and sociology. The questions and problems they study emerge from traditions within those disciplines. Each discipline is organized around attention to basic questions and the research within that discipline derives from concern about those basic questions. In Table 5.1 examples of fundamental questions in three disciplines are listed.

There are many disciplines, each with its own fundamental questions. The basic questions of each discipline flow from the basic concerns and traditions of that discipline. Researchers working within any specific disciplinary tradition strive to make a contribution to knowledge in that discipline and thereby contribute to answering the fundamental questions of the discipline. The most prestigious contribution to knowledge takes the form of a *theory* that explains the phenomenon under investigation. Basic researchers work to generate new theories or test existing theories. Doctoral students are typically expected to make theoretical contributions in their dissertations. Theories encapsulate the knowledge of a discipline.

The findings of basic research are published in scholarly books, journals and dissertations. Each discipline has its own traditions, norms, and rules for deciding what constitutes valid research in that discipline. To be published within the major journals of any particular discipline, scientists must engage in the

Table 5.1
Fundamental Disciplinary Questions

Discipline	Basic Questions
Anthropology	What is the nature of culture? How does culture emerge? How is it transmitted? What are the functions of culture?
Psychology	Why do individuals behave as they do? How do human beings behave, think, feel, and know?
Sociology	What holds groups and societies together? How do various forms of social organization emerge and what are their functions? What are the structures and processes of human social organizations?

Table 5.2
Applied Research Questions

Applied Research Field	Illustrative Problems to be studied
Applied Anthropology	How can the culture of a small minority group be preserved when that group is engulfed by a larger or more powerful people with a different culture?
Applied Psychology	How can individuals become aware of, take control of, and change dysfunctional attitudes and behaviors?
Applied Sociology	How can people of different races, religions, or socio-economic statuses live and work together productively within a community?

kind of research that is valued by the researchers in that disciplinary tradition.

Qualitative inquiry contributes to basic research through "grounded theory" (Glaser and Strauss, 1967), essentially an inductive strategy for generating and confirming theory that emerges from close involvement and direct contact with the empirical world. Chapter 3 reviewed theoretical traditions closely associated with qualitative inquiry, for example, ethnography and phenomenology

Basic qualitative research typically requires a relatively lengthy and intensive period of fieldwork. The rigor of field techniques will be subject to peer review. Particular attention must be given to the accuracy, validity and integrity of the results.

Applied Research

Applied researchers work on human problems. The purpose of the research is to contribute knowledge that will help people understand the nature of a problem so that human beings can more effectively control their environment. While in basic research the source of questions is the traditions within a scholarly discipline, in applied research the source of questions is in the problems and concerns experienced by people. The purpose of applied research, then, is to generate potential solutions to human and societal problems.

Applied researchers take the findings, understandings, and explanations of basic research and *apply* them to real-world problems and experiences. This means that the applied researcher searches for applications of basic disciplinary knowledge to real-world problems.

The results of applied research arc published in journals that specialize in applied research within the traditions of a problem area or a discipline.

In Table 5.2 examples are provided of applied research questions for each of the disciplines listed previously. Notice the difference between these questions and the questions being asked by basic researchers. The difference is that applied researchers are trying to understand how to deal with a problem while basic researchers are trying to understand and explain the basic nature of some phenomenon.

Applied research concerns have also given rise to a variety of interdisciplinary fields. For example, work on environmental studies often involves researchers from a number of disciplines. In agricultural research, the field of integrated pest management (IPM) includes researchers from entomology, agronomy, agricultural economics, and horticulture. Fields of interdisciplinary research in the social sciences include gerontology, criminal justice studies, women's studies, and family research. These are problem areas for applied research rather than disciplines in which one would undertake basic research.

Applied qualitative researchers are able to bring their personal insights and experiences into any recommendations that may emerge. Audiences for applied research are often not clear. Time lines depend a great deal on the timeliness and urgency of a problem if the results are actually to be applied.

Evaluation Research: Summative and Formative

Once solutions to problems are identified, policies and programs are designed to intervene in society and bring about change. Hopefully, the intervention and changes will be effective in helping to solve problems. However, the effectiveness of any given human intervention is a matter subject to study. Thus the next point on the research continuum is the conduct of evaluation and policy research to test out the effectiveness of specific solutions and human interventions.

While applied research seeks to understand societal problems and identify potential solutions, evaluation research studies the processes and outcomes aimed at attempted solutions. Evaluators study programs, policies, personnel, organizations and products. Evaluation research can be conducted on virtually any explicit attempt to solve problems or bring about planned change.

As we examine the research continuum, it is helpful to distinguish two quite different purposes for evaluation. Evaluators distinguish summative' evaluations from "formative" evaluations (Herman et al., 1987). Summative evaluations serve the purpose of rendering an overall judgment about the effectiveness of a program, policy or product for the purpose of saying that *the idea itself* is or is not effective and, therefore, has the potential of being generalizable to other situations. Summative evaluations, then, examine and study specific programs, policies, and products in order to generalize about the effectiveness of the human action under investigation. The "generalization" may take the form of deciding that a program should be continued; it may lead to a decision to expand a pilot program to new sites; or it may lead to program or policy termination. Summative evaluations seldom rely entirely, or even primarily, on qualitative data because of

the interest in controlled comparisons, generalization, and relatively larger samples. Summative evaluation research tests the effectiveness of some human intervention or action (or the purpose of deciding if that program or policy is effective within its limited context *and* under what conditions it is likely to be effective in other situations or places.

Formative evaluation, on the other hand, is limited entirely to a focus on a specific context. Formative evaluation serves the purpose of improving a specific program, policy, group of staff (in a personnel evaluation), or product. Formative evaluations aim at "forming" the thing being studied. Formative evaluators want to help improve human endeavors. There is no attempt in formative evaluation to generalize findings beyond the setting in which one is working. The purpose of the research is to improve effectiveness within that setting. Formative evaluations rely heavily on process studies, implementation evaluations, case studies and evaluability assessments (see Chapter 4). Formative evaluations often rely heavily, even primarily, on qualitative methods.

Formative and summative evaluations involve fundamental and very important distinctions that speak to the heart of variations in research purposes: the extent to which one seeks to generalize. Basic researchers are interested in formulating and testing theoretical constructs and propositions that ideally generalize across time and space. The most powerful kinds of findings in basic science are those findings that are universal. Basic researchers, then, are searching for fundamental patterns of the universe, the earth, nature, society, and human beings.

Applied researchers seek more limited generalizations. Applied research findings typically are limited to a specific time, place, and condition. For example, a researcher studying the nature of family problems in the 1980s would not expect those problems to be the same as families experienced in the 1880s. While the research might include making such comparisons, applied researchers understand that problems emerge within particular time and space boundaries. Summative evaluation researchers are seeking still more limited generalizations. Their generalizations concern the effectiveness of specific interventions on specified populations under specifiable conditions. However this still permits the researcher to seek patterns that cut across programs or policies in a number of different places and for a number of different groups.

Formative evaluation does not seek to generalize at all beyond the specific intervention being studied. The purpose of formative evaluation is to improve human intervention within a specific set of activities at a specific time for a specific group of people.

Action Research

The final point on the continuum is action research. Action research aims at solving specific problems within a program, organization, or community. Action research explicitly and purposefully becomes part of the change process by engaging the people in the program or organization in studying their own problems in order to solve those problems (Whyte, 1989). As a result, the distinction between research and action becomes quite blurred and the research methods tend to be less Systematic, more informal, and quite specific to the problem, people, and organization for which the research is undertaken.

Both formative evaluation and action research focus on specific programs at specific points in time. There is no intention, typically, to generalize beyond those specific settings. The difference between formative evaluation and action research centers on the extent to which the research is systematic, the different kinds of problems studied, and the extent to which there is a special role for the researcher as distinct from the people being researched.

In formative evaluation there is a formal design and the data are collected by a researcher. The focus of formative research is on ways of improving the effectiveness of a program, a policy, an organization a product, or a staff unit. In action research design and data collection tend to be more informal, the people in the situation are often directly involved in gathering the information and then studying themselves, and the results are used internally to attack specific problems within a program, organization, or community. While action research may be used as part of an overall organization or community develop ment process, it most typically would focus on specific problems and issues within the organization or community rather than on the overall effectiveness of an entire program or organization. Rapid reconnaissance qualitative studies, as described in Chapter 4, are a type of action research that may be used to formulate a more formal applied research design. Thus, along this research continuum, action research has the most narrow focus.

The findings of formative evaluation and action research are seldom disseminated beyond the immediate program or organization within which the study takes place. In many instances, there may not even be a full written research report. Publication and dissemination of findings are more likely to be through briefings, staff discussions, and oral communications. Summaries of findings and recommendations will be distributed for discussion, but the formality of the reporting and the nature of the research publications are quite different from basic, applied, or even summative evaluation research.

The Purpose of Purpose Distinctions

There are not hard-and-fast lines of demarcation between these five different types of research. The continuum ranges from very basic, long-term research aimed at theory development and knowledge for its own sake to highly action-oriented research aimed at solving immediate problems in as short a time as possible. It is important to understand variations in purpose along this continuum because different purposes typically lead to different ways of conceptualizing problems, different

designs, different types of data gathering, and different ways of publicizing and disseminating findings.

Another reason it is important to understand the variations along the continuum is that researchers engaged in research at various points along the continuum, have very strong opinions and feelings about researchers at other points along the continuum. Research can be a highly political activity that generates opposing opinions and strong emotions. Basic and applied researchers, for example, would often dispute even calling formative and action research by the name research. The standards that basic researchers apply to what they would consider "good" research excludes even some applied research because it may not manifest the conceptual clarity and theoretical rigor in real-world situations that basic researchers value. Formative and action researchers, on the other hand, may attack basic research for being esoteric and irrelevant.

Debates about the meaningfulness, rigor, significance, and relevance of various approaches to research are regular features of university life. On the whole, within universities and among scholars, the status hierarchy in science attributes the highest status to basic research, secondary status to applied research, little status to summative evaluation research, and virtually no status to formative and action research. The status hierarchy is reversed in real-world settings, where people with problems attribute the greatest significance to action and formative research that can help them solve their problems in a timely way and attach the least importance to basic research, which they consider remote and largely irrelevant to what they are doing on a day-to-day basis.

The distinctions along the continuum are not only distinctions about purpose and how one conducts research, but they also involve the issue of what one calls what one does. In other words, a person conducting basic research for the purpose of contributing to theory within a discipline may find it helpful to call that work "applied research" in order to get certain kinds of funding. Summative evaluation researchers may describe what they are doing as "formative evaluation" in order to make their work more acceptable to program staff resistant to being studied. On the other hand, applied researchers may call what they are doing "basic research" in order to increase its acceptability among scholars.

In short, there are no clear lines dividing the points along the continuum. Part of what determines where a particular kind of research falls along the continuum is how the researcher describes what is being done and its purpose. Different reviewers of the same piece of research might well use a different label to describe it. What is important for our purposes is that researchers understand the implications of these distinctions, the choices involved, and the implications of those choices for both the kind of research to be undertaken and one's status as a professional within various social groups.

Table 5.3 summarizes some of the major differences among the different kinds of research.

Table 5.3

A Typology of Research Purposes

Types of Research	Purpose	Focus of Research	Desired Results	Desired Level of Generalization	Key Assumptions	Publication Mode	Standard for Judging
Basic research	Knowledge as an end in itself; discover truth.	Questions deemed important by one's discipline or personal intellectual interest.	Contribution to theory	Across time and space (ideal)	The world is patterned; those patterns are knowable and explainable.	Major refereed scholarly journals in one's discipline, scholarly books	Rigor of research, universality and verifiability of theory
Applied research	Understand the nature and sources of human and societal problems.	Questions deemed important by society.	Contributions to theories that can be used to formulate problem-solving programs and interventions	Within as general a time and space as possible, but clearly limited application context	Human and societal problems can be understood and solved with knowledge.	Specialized academic journals, applied research journals within disciplines, interdisciplinary problem-focused journals	Rigor and theoretical insight into the
Summative evaluation	Determine effectiveness of human interventions and actions (programs, policies, personnel products).	Goals of the intervention.	Judgments and generalizations about effective types of interventions and the conditions under which those efforts are effective	All interventions with similar goals	What works one place under specified conditions should work elsewhere.	Evaluation reports for program funders and policymakers, specialized journals	Generalizability to future efforts and to other programs and policy issues
Formative evaluation	Improving an intervention: a program, policy, organization, or product.	Strengths and weaknesses of the specific program, policy product, or personnel being studied.	Recommendations for improvements	Limited to specific setting studied	People can and will use information to improve what they're doing.	Oral briefings; conferences; internal report; limited circulation to similar programs, other evaluators	Usefulness to and actual use by intended users in the setting studied
Action research	Solve problems in a program, organization, or community.	Organization and community problems.	Immediate action; solving problems as quickly as possible	Here and now	People in a setting can solve problems by studying themselves.	Interpersonal interactions among research participants; informal, unpublished	Feelings about the process among research participants, feasibility of the solution generated

EXAMPLES OF DIFFERENT TYPES OF RESEARCH QUESTIONS

To further clarify these distinctions, it may be helpful to take a particular issue and look at how that issue would be approached for each type of research.

A Family Research Example

Social and behavioral scientists are interested, among other things, in families. Let us examine the different kinds of questions that can be asked about families for different research purposes (see Table 5.4). All of the research examples in Table 5.4 focus on families, but the purpose of each type of research and the questions asked are quite different. With clarity about purpose, it is possible to begin considering specific design alternatives and strategies. Clarity about purpose helps in making decisions about critical trade-offs in evaluation research designs.

Table 5.4
Research Examples

Basic research	What are the variations in types of families and what functions do those variations serve?
Applied research	What is the divorce rate among different kinds of families in the United States and what explains different rates of divorce among different groups?
Summative evaluation research	What is the effectiveness of a federal- and state-funded educational research teaching family members communication skills?
Formative evaluation research	How can the communication program teaching family coping skills be improved? What are the program's strengths and weaknesses?
Action research	A self-study by family members in a particular church, organization. or community to figure how they can be more supportive of and help each other.

CRITRICAL TRADE-OFFS IN EVALUATION DESIGN

Purposes, strategies, and trade-offs – these themes go together. A discussion of design strategies and trade-offs is necessitated by the fact that *there are no perfect research designs*. There are always trade-offs. These trade-offs are necessitated by limited resources, limited time, and limits on the human ability to grasp the complex nature of social reality.

The very first trade-offs come in framing the research or evaluation questions to be studied. The problem here is to determine the extent to which it is desirable to study one or a few questions in great depth or to study many questions but in less depth. This is what Guba (1978) calls the "boundary problem" in naturalistic inquiry evaluation. Once a potential set of evaluation questions has been generated, it is necessary to begin the process of prioritizing those questions in order to decide which of them ought to be pursued at a particular point in time. Should all parts of the program be studied or only certain parts? Should all clients be studied or only some subset of clients? Should the evaluator aim at describing all program processes or is there reason to examine only certain selected processes in depth? Should all outcomes be examined or should the evaluation focus upon the attainment of only certain outcomes of particular interest at this point in time? These are questions that are discussed and negotiated with intended users of the evaluation. In basic research these questions are answered by the nature of the theoretical contribution to be made. But

in evaluation and action research, the information needs of intended users are the primary basis for determining focus.

In my own experience, the problem of establishing focus and priorities is much more difficult than the problem of generating potential questions at the beginning of the evaluation. Once a group of intended evaluation users begins to take seriously the notion that they can learn from the collection and analysis of evaluative information, they soon find that there are lots of things they would like to find out. The evaluator's role is to help them move from a rather extensive list of potential questions to a much shorter list of realistically possible questions and finally to a focused list of *essential and necessary questions*.

Review of relevant literature can also help focus the study. It is helpful to find out how others have approached similar concerns. Yet, reviewing the literature can present a quandary in qualitative inquiry because it may bias the researcher's thinking and reduce openness to whatever emerges in the field. Thus a literature review may not take place until after data collection. Alternatively, the literature review may go on simultaneously with fieldwork, permitting a creative interplay among the processes of data collection, literature review, and researcher introspection (see Marshall and Rossman, 1989:38-40). There are trade-offs, advantages, and disadvantages related to when to review the literature: before, during, or after fieldwork- or on a continual basis throughout the study.

An example of variations in evaluation focus may help illustrate the kinds of trade-offs involved in designing a study. Suppose that a group of educators is interested in studying how a school program affects the social development of school-age children. They want to know how the interactions of children with others in the school program contribute to the development of social skills. They believe that those social skills will be different for different children, and they are not sure of the range of social interactions that may occur, so they are interested in a qualitative inquiry evaluation that will capture variations in program experience and individualized outcomes. Still, there are trade-offs in determining the final focus.

It is clear that any given child has social interactions with a great many people. The problem in focusing our evaluation research endeavor is to determine how much of the social reality experienced by children we should attempt to describe. In a narrowly focused evaluation we might select one particular set of interactions and limit our study to those interactions – for example, the social interactions between teachers and children. Broadening the scope somewhat, we might decide to look at only those interactions that occur in the classroom, thereby increasing the scope of the study to include interactions not only between teacher and child but also among peers in the classroom and between any volunteers and visitors to the classroom and the children. Broadening the scope of the study still more, we might decide to look at all of the social relationships that children experience in schools; in this case we would move beyond the classroom to look at interactions with other teaching personnel in the school – for example, the librarian, school counselors, special subject teachers, the custodian, and/or school administrative staff. Broadening the scope of the study still further, the educators might decide that it is important to look at the social relationships children experience at home and at school in order to understand how children experience those settings differently to better understand the unique effects of the school. In this case we would include in our design interactions with parents, siblings, and other people in the home. Finally, one might look at the social relationships experienced throughout the full range of societal contacts that children have, including church, clubs, and even mass media contacts.

All of these are potentially important evaluation research questions. Suppose that we have a set amount of resources – for example, $25,000 – to conduct a study. At some level, any of these research endeavors could be undertaken for $25,000. It is immediately clear, however, that *there is a trade-off betweeen breadth and depth.* A highly focused question like the interactions between teacher and child could consume the entire amount of our resources and allow us to investigate the problem in great depth. On the other hand, we might attempt to look at all social relationships that children experience, but to look at each of them in a relatively cursory way in order, perhaps, to explore which of those relationships is primary. (if school relationships have very little impact on social development in comparison with relationships outside the school, policymakers could use that information to decide whether the school program ought to be redesigned to have greater impact on social development or, alternatively, if the school should forget about trying to directly affect social development at all.) *The trade-offs involved are the classic trade-offs between breath and depth.*

Breadth Versus Depth

In many ways a major trade-off between quantitative methods and qualitative methods is a trade-off between breadth and depth. Qualitative methods permit the evaluation researcher to study selected issues in depth and detail; the fact that data collection is not constrained by predetermined categories of analysis contributes to the depth and detail of qualitative data. Quantitative methods, on the other hand, require the use of a standardized approach so that the experiences of people are limited to certain predetermined response categories. The advantage of the quantitative approach is that it is possible to measure the reactions of many subjects to a limited set of questions, thus facilitating comparison and statistical aggregation of the data. By contrast, qualitative methods typically produce a wealth of detailed data about a much smaller number of people and cases.

The breadth versus depth trade-off is applicable not only in comparing quantitative and qualitative methods; the same trade-off applies within qualitative methods. The human relations specialists tell us that we can never *fully* understand the experience of another person. The design issue is how much time and effort we are willing to invest in trying to increase our understanding about any single person's experience.

Again, under conditions of limited resources, we can look at a narrow range of experiences for a larger number of people or a broader range of experiences for a smaller number of people. Take the case of interviews. Interviewing with an instrument that provides a respondent with largely open-ended stimuli typically takes a great deal of time. In North Dakota when I was studying various aspects of open education we developed an open-ended interview consisting of 20 questions that were asked of children in grades one to eight in various open classrooms. Those questions consisted of items such as, "What do you like most about school?" and "What don't you like about school?" These interviews took between half an hour and two hours depending on how articulate students were and how old they were. It would certainly have been possible to have longer interviews. Indeed, I have conducted in-depth interviews with people that ran six to sixteen hours over a period of a couple of days. On the other hand, it would have been possible to ask fewer questions, to make the interviews shorter, and to obtain less depth.

To further illustrate this trade-off between breadth and depth in sampling human behavior, let us consider another example of the full range of possibilities. It is possible (and indeed it has been done) to study a single individual over an extended period of time-for example, the study, in depth, of one week in the life of one child. This necessitates gathering detailed information about every occurrence in that child's life and every interaction involving that child during some time period. With a more narrow research question we might study several children during a more limited period of time. With a still more limited focused question, or an interview of a half hour, we could interview yet a larger number of children on a smaller number of issues. The extreme case would be to spend all of our resources and time asking a single question of as many children as we could interview given the resource constraints.

There is no rule of thumb that tells a researcher precisely how to focus a study. The extent to which a research question is broad or narrow depends on purpose, the resources available, the time available, and the interests of those involved. In brief, these are not choices between good and bad, but choices among alternatives, all of which have merit.

Units of Analysis

The evaluation design specifies the unit or units of analysis to be studied. Decisions about samples, both sample size and sampling strategies, depend on prior decisions about the appropriate unit of analysis to study.

Sometimes individual people, clients, or students are the unit of analysis. This means that the primary focus of data collection will be on what is happening to individuals in a setting and how individuals are affected by the setting. Individual variation would be the primary qualitative research issue.

Comparing groups of people in a program or across programs involves a different unit of analysis. One may be interested in comparing demographic groups (males compared with females, whites compared with blacks) or programmatic groups (dropouts versus people who complete the program, people who do well versus people who do poorly, people who experience group therapy versus people who experience individual therapy). One or more groups are selected as the unit of analysis when there is some important characteristic that separates people into groups and when that characteristic has important implications for the program.

A different unit of analysis involves focusing on different parts of a program. Different classrooms within a school might be studied, making the classroom the unit of analysis. Outpatient and inpatient programs in a medical facility might be studied. The intake part of a program might be studied separately from the service delivery part of a program as separate units of analysis. Entire programs can become the unit of analysis. In state and national programs where there are a number of local sites, the appropriate unit of analysis may be local projects. The focus in this case would be on variations among project sites more than on variations among individuals within projects.

These different units of analysis are not mutually exclusive. However, each unit of analysis implies a different kind of data collection, a different focus for the analysis of data, and a different level at which statements about findings and conclusions would be made. Neighborhoods can be units of analysis or communities, cities, states, and even nations in the case of international programs.

One of the strengths of qualitative analysis is looking at program units holistically. This means doing more than aggregating data from individuals to get overall program results. When a program, group, or community is the unit of analysis, qualitative methods involve observations and description focused directly on that unit.

In qualitative studies, units of analysis may also be particular kinds of events, occurrences, or incidents. For example, a quality assurance effort in a health or mental health program might focus only on those critical incidents in which a patient fails to receive expected or desirable treatment. A criminal justice evaluation could focus on violent events or instances in which juveniles run away from treatment.

Time sampling (sampling periods or units of time) can be an especially important approach because programs may function in different ways at different times during the year. Of course, with some programs there is never a good time to collect data. I have learned that this is the case with schools. Educators will tell you

that you don't want to collect data in the schools before Halloween because the school year is just getting started and the kids aren't quite fixed in the patterns that will be maintained later in the year. The period between Halloween and Thanksgiving is really too short to do very much, and, then, of course, after Thanksgiving everybody's getting ready for Christmas, so that's not a typical or convenient period. It then takes students a few weeks after Christmas to get their attention focused back on school and then the winter malaise sets in and both teachers and students become deeply depressed with the endlessness of winter (at least in Minnesota). Then, of course, once spring hits, attention is focused on the close of school and the kids want to be outside, so that's not an effective time to gather data.

There are limits to how much one can apply logic and deduction in making sampling decisions, whether the decision is about which time periods to sample or which activities to observe. The trick is to keep coming back to the criterion of usefulness. What data collected during what time period describing what activities would make a difference? There are no perfect evaluation designs, only more and less useful ones.

The key issue in selecting and making decisions about the appropriate unit of analysis is to decide what it is you want to be able to say something about at the end of the study. Do you want to have findings about individuals, families, groups, or some other unit of analysis? At what level do decision makers really need information? Do they want information about the different experiences of individuals in programs or do they want to know about variations in program processes at different sites? These are differences in focus that are critical to the design but may not be easy to determine. The decision maker typically will be unable to say to the evaluator, "The unit of analysis we want to study is _____." The evaluator must be able to hear the real issues involved in the decision maker's questions and translate those issues into the appropriate unit of analysis, then check out that translation with the intended evaluation users.

PURPOSEFUL SAMPLING

Perhaps nothing better captures the difference between quantitative and qualitative methods than the different logics that undergird sampling approaches. Qualitative inquiry typically focuses in depth on relatively small samples, even single cases ($n = 1$), selected purposefully. Quantitative methods typically depend on larger samples selected randomly. Not only are the techniques for sampling different, but the very logic of each approach is unique because the purpose of each strategy is different.

The logic and power of probability sampling depends on selecting a truly random and statistically representative sample that will permit confident generalization from the sample to a larger population. The purpose is generalization.

The logic and power of purposeful sampling lies in selecting information-rich cases for study in depth. Information-rich cases are those from which one can learn a great deal about issues of central importance to the purpose of the research, thus the term purposeful sampling. For example, if the purpose of an evaluation is to increase the effectiveness of a program in reaching lower-socioeconomic groups, one may learn a great deal more by focusing in depth on understanding the needs, interests, and incentives of a small number of carefully selected poor families than by gathering standardized information from a large, statistically representative sample of the whole program. The purpose of purposeful sampling is to select information-rich cases whose study will illuminate the questions under study.

There are several different strategies for purposefully selecting information-rich cases. The logic of each strategy serves a particular evaluation purpose.

(1) Extreme or deviant case sampling. This approach focuses on cases that are rich in information because they are unusual or special in some way. Unusual or special cases may be particularly troublesome or especially enlightening, such as outstanding successes or notable failures. If, for example, the evaluation was aimed at gathering data to help a national program reach more clients, one might compare a few project sites that have long waiting lists with those that have short waiting lists. If staff morale was an issue, one might study and compare high-morale programs to low-morale programs.

The logic of extreme case sampling is that lessons may be learned about unusual conditions or extreme outcomes that are relevant to improving more typical programs. Let's suppose that we are interested in studying a national program with hundreds of local sites. We know that many programs are operating reasonably well, even quite well, and that other programs verge on being disasters. We also know that most programs are doing "okay." This information comes from knowledgeable sources who have made site visits to enough programs to have a basic idea about what the variation is. The question is this: How should programs be sampled for the study? If one wanted to precisely document the natural variation among programs, a random sample would be appropriate, preferably a random sample of sufficient size to be truly representative of and permit generalization: to the total population of programs. However, some information is already available on what program variation is like. The question of more immediate interest may concern extreme cases. With limited resources and limited time an evaluator might learn more by intensively studying one or more examples of really poor programs and one or more examples of really excellent programs. The evaluation focus, then, becomes a question of understanding under what conditions programs get into trouble and under what conditions programs exemplify excellence. It is not even necessary to randomly sample poor programs or excellent programs. The researchers and intended users involved in the study think through *what cases they could learn the most from* and those are the cases that are selected for study.

In a single program the same strategy may apply. Instead of studying some representative sample of people in the setting, the evaluator may focus on studying and understanding selected cases of special interest, for example, unexpected dropouts or outstanding successes. in many instances more can be learned from intensively studying extreme or unusual cases than can be learned from statistical depictions of what the average case is like. In other evaluations detailed information about special cases can be used to supplement statistical data about the normal distribution of participants.

Ethnomethodologists use a form of extreme case sampling when they do their field experiments. Ethnomethodologists are interested in everyday experiences of routine living that depend on deeply understood, shared understandings among people in a setting (see Chapter 3). One way of exposing these implicit assumptions and norms on which everyday life is based is to create disturbances that deviate from the norm. Observing the reactions to someone eating like a pig in a restaurant and then interviewing people about what they saw and how they felt would be an example of studying a deviant sample to illuminate the ordinary, The Peters and Waterman (1982) best-selling study of "America's best run companies," *In Search of Excellence*, exemplifies the logic of purposeful, extreme group sampling. Their study was based on a sample of 62 companies "never intended to be perfectly representative of U.S. industry as a whole . . . [but] a list of companies considered to be innovative and excellent by an informed group of observers of the business scene" (Peters and Waterman, 1982: 19).

Another excellent example of extreme group sampling is Angela Browne's (1987) study, *When Battered Women Kill.* She conducted in-depth studies of the most extreme cases of domestic violence to elucidate The phenomenon of battering and abuse. The extreme nature of the cases presented are what render them so powerful. Browne's book is an exemplar of qualitative inquiry using purposeful sampling for applied research.

(2) Intensity sampling. Intensity sampling involves the same logic as extreme case sampling but with less emphasis on the extremes. An intensity sample consists of information-rich cases that manifest the phenomenon of interest intensely (but not extremely). Extreme or deviant cases may be so unusual as to distort the manifestation of the phenomenon of interest. Using the logic of intensity sampling, one seeks excellent or rich examples of the phenomenon of interest, but not unusual cases.

Heuristic research uses intensity sampling. Heuristic research draws explicitly on the intense personal experiences of the researcher, for example, experiences with loneliness or jealousy. Coresearchers who have experienced these phenomena intensely also participate in the study (see Chapter 3). The heuristic researcher is not typically seeking pathological or extreme manifestations of loneliness, jealousy, or whatever phenomenon is of interest. Such extreme cases might not lend themselves to the reflective process of heuristic inquiry On the other hand, if the experience of the heuristic researcher and his or her coresearchers is quite mild, there won't be much to study. Thus the researcher seeks a sample of sufficient intensity to elucidate the phenomenon of interest.

The same logic applies in a program evaluation. Extreme successes or unusual failures may be discredited as being too extreme or unusual for gaining information. Therefore, the evaluator may select cases that manifest sufficient intensity to illuminate the nature of success or failure, but not at the extreme.

Intensity sampling involves some prior information and considerable judgment. The researcher must do some exploratory work to determine the nature of the variation in the situation understudy. One can then sample intense examples of the phenomenon of interest.

(3) Maximum variation, sampling. This strategy for purposeful sampling aims at capturing and describing the central themes or principal outcomes that cut across a great deal of participant or program variation. For small samples a great deal of heterogeneity can be a problem because individual cases are so different from each other. The maximim variation sampling strategy turns, that apparent weakness into a strength by applying the following logic: Any common patterns that emerge from great variation are of particular interest and value in capturing the core experiences and central, shared aspects or impact of a program.

How does one maximize variation in a small sample? One begins by identifying diverse characteristics or criteria for constructing the sample. Suppose a statewide program has project sites spread around the state, some in rural areas, some in urban areas, and some in suburban areas. The evaluation lacks sufficient resources to randomly select enough project sites to generalize across the state. The evaluator can at least be sure that the geographical variation among sites is represented in the study.

When selecting a small sample of great diversity, the data colection and analysis will yield two kinds of findings: (1) high-quality, detailed descriptions of each case, which are useful for documenting uniqueness, and (2) important shared patterns that cut across cases and derive their significance from having emerged out of heterogeneity.

The same strategy can be used within a single program inselecting individuals for study. By including in the sample individuals the evaluator determines have had quite different experiences, it is possible to more thoroughly describe the variation in the group and to understand variations in experiences while also investigating core elements and shared outcomes. The evaluator using a *maximum variation sampling strategy* would not be attempting to generalize findings to all people or all groups but would be looking for information that elucidates programmatic variation and significant common patterns within that variation.

(4) Homogeneous samples. In direct contrast to maximum variation sampling is the strategy of picking a small homogeneous sample. The purpose here is to describe some particular subgroup in depth. A program that has many different kinds of participants may need indepth information about a particular subgroup. For example, a parent education program that involves many different kinds of parents may focus a qualitative evaluation on the experiences of single-parent female heads of household because that is a particularly difficult group to reach and hold in the program.

Focus group interviews are typically based on homogeneous groups. Focus group interviews involve conducting open-ended interviews with groups of five to eight people on specially targeted or focused issues. The use of focus groups in evaluation will be discussed at greater length in the chapter on interviewing. The point here is that sampling for focus groups typically involves bringing together people of similar backgrounds and experiences to participate in a group interview about major program issues that affect them.

(5) Typical case sampling. In describing a program or its participants to people not familiar with the program it can be helpful to provide a qualitative profile of one or more "typical" cases. These cases are selected with the cooperation of key informants, such as program staff or knowledgeable participants, who can help identify what is typical. It is also possible to select typical cases from survey data, a demographic analysis of averages, or other programmatic data that provide a normal distribution of characteristics from which to identify "average" examples. Keep in mind that the purpose of a qualitative profile of one or more typical cases is to describe and illustrate what is typical to those unfamiliar with the programnot to make generalized statements about the experiences of all participants. The sample is illustrative not definitive.

When entire programs or communities are the unit of analysis, it is also possible to sample somewhat typical cases. Again, the study of such typical programs does not, of course, permit generalizations in any rigorous sense. It does, however, mean that the processes and effects described for the typical program need not be dismissed as peculiar to "poor" sites or "excellent" sites. When the typical site sampling strategy is used, the site is specifically selected because it is not in any major way atypical, extreme, deviant, or intensely unusual. This strategy is often appropriate in sampling villages for community development studies in Third World countries. A study of a typical village illuminates key issues that must be considered in any development project aimed at this kind of village.

Decision makers may have made their peace with the fact that there will always be some poor programs and some excellent programs, but the programs they really want more information about are those run-of-the-mill programs that are "hard to get a handle on". It is important, when using this strategy, to attempt to get broad consensus about which programs are "typical." If a number of such programs are identified, only a few can be studied, and there is no other basis for selecting among them purposefully then it is possible to randomly select from among all "typical" programs identified to select those few typical cases that actually will be included in the study.

(6) Stratified purposeful sampling. It is also clearly possible to combine a typical case sampling strategy with others, essentially taking *a stratified purposeful sample* of above average, average, and below average cases. This is less than a full maximum variation sample. The purpose of a stratified purposeful sample is to capture major variations rather than to identify a common core, although the latter may also emerge in the analysis. Each of the strata would constitute a fairly homogeneous sample. This strategy differs from stratified random sampling in that the sample sizes are likely to be too small for generalization or statistical representativeness.

(7) Critical case sampling. Another strategy for selecting purposeful samples is to look for critical cases. Critical cases are those that can make a point quite dramatically or are, for some reason, particularly important in the scheme of things A clue to the existence of a critical case is a statement to the effect that "if it happens there, it will happen anywhere," or, vice versa, "if it doesn't happen there, it won't happen anywhere." The focus of the data gathering in this instance is on understanding what is happening in that critical case. Another clue to the existence of a critical case is a key informant observation to the effect that "if that group is having problem then we can be sure all the groups are having problems."

Looking for the critical case is particularly important where resources may limit the evaluation to the study of only a single site. Under such conditions it makes strategic sense to pick the site that would yield the most information and have the greatest impact on the development of knowledge. While studying one or a few critical cases does not technically permit broad generalizations to all possible cases, *logical generalizations* can often be made from the weight of evidence produced in studying a single, critical case,

Physics provides a good example of such a critical case. In Galileo's study of gravity he wanted to find out if the weight of an object affected the rate of speed at which it would fall. Rather than randomly sampling objects of different weights in order to generalize to all objects in the world, he selected a critical case – the feather. If in a vacuum, as he demonstrated, a feather fell at the same rate as some heavier object (a coin), then he could logically generalize from this one critical case to all objects. His findings were enormously useful and credible.

There are many comparable critical cases in social science research – if one is creative in looking for them. For example, suppose national policymakers want to get local communities involved in makng decisions about how their local program will be run, but they aren't sure that the communities will understand the complex regulations governing their involvement. The first critical case is to evaluate the regulations in a community of well-educated citizens; if they can't

understand the regulations, then less-educated folks are sure to find the regulations incomprehensible. Or conversely, one might consider the critical case to be a community consisting of people with quite low levels of education: "If they can understand the regulations, anyone can."

Identification of critical cases depends on recognition of the key dimensions that make for a critical case. A critical case might be indicated by the financial state of a program; a program with particularly high or particularly low cost-per-client ratios might suggest a critical case. A critical case might come from a particularly difficult program location. If the funders of a new program are worried about recruiting clients or participants into a program, it may make sense to study the site where resistance to the program is expected to be greatest to provide the most rigorous test of the possibility of program recruitment. If the program works in that site, "It could work anywhere."

World-renowned medical hypnotist Milton H. Erickson became a critical case in the field of hypnosis. Erickson was so skillful that he became widely known for "his ability to succeed with "impossibles" – people who have exhausted the traditional medical, dental, psycho-therapeutic, hypnotic and religious avenues for assisting them in their need, and have not been able to make the changes they desire" (Grinder et al., 1977: 109), If Milton Erickson couldn't help, no one could help. He was able to demonstrate that anyone could be hypnotized.

(8) Snowball or chain sampling. This is an approach for locating information-rich key informants or critical cases. The process begins by asking well-situated people: "Who knows a lot about _____? Who should I talk to?" By asking a number of people who else to talk with, the snowball gets bigger and bigger as you accumulate new information-rich cases. In most programs or systems, a few key names or incidents are mentioned repeatedly. Those people or events recommended as valuable by a number of different informants take on special importance. The chain of recommended informants will typically diverge initially as many possible sources are recommended, then converge as a few key names get mentioned over and over.

The Peters and Waterman (1982) study *In Search of Excellence* began with snowball sampling, asking a broad group of knowledgeable people to identify well-run companies. Another excellent and well-known example was Rosabeth Moss Kanter's (1983) study of innovation reported in *The Change Masters*. Her book focused on ten core case studies. She began her search for the "best' or "most innovative" companies by getting the views of corporate experts in human resource fields. Nominations for cases to study snowballed from there and then converged into a small number of core cases nominated by a number of different informants.

(9) Criterion sampling. The logic of criterion sampling is to review and study all cases that meet some predetermined criterion of importance. This approach is

common in quality assurance efforts. For example, the expected range of participation in a mental health outpatient program might be 4 to 26 weeks. All cases that exceed 28 weeks are reviewed and studied to find out what is happening and to make sure the case is being appropriately handled.

Critical incidents can be a source of criterion sampling. For example, all incidents of client abuse in a program may be objects of in-depth evaluation in a quality assurance effort. All former mental health clients who commit suicide within three months of release may constitute a sample for in-depth, qualitative study. In a school setting, all students who are absent more than half the time may merit the in-depth attention of a qualitative case study The point of criterion sampling is to be sure to understand cases that are likely to be information rich because they may reveal major system weaknesses that become targets of opportunity for program or system improvement.

Criterion sampling can add an important qualitative component to a management information system or an ongoing program monitoring system. All cases in the data system that exhibit certain predetermined criterion characteristics are routinely identified for in-depth, qualitative analysis. Criterion sampling also can be applied to identify cases from quantitative questionnaire or tests for in-depth follow-up.

(10) Theory-based or operatiotial construct sampling. A more formal basic research version of criterion sampling is theory based sampling. The researcher samples incidents, slices of life, time periods, or people on the basis of their potential manifestation or representation of important theoretical constructs. The sample becomes, by definition, representative of the phenomenon of interest. An ecological psychologist (see Chapter 3) is interested, for example, in studying the interaction between a person and the environment. Instances of such interaction must be defined based on theoretical premises in order to study examples that represent the phenomenon of interest.

This differs from the more practical sampling in program evaluation. The evaluator doesn't need a theory-based definition of "program" because the entity to be studied is usually legally or financially defined. However to sample social science phenomena that represent theoretical constructs of interest, one must define the construct to be sampled, such as person-environmental interactions or instances of social deviance, identity crisis, creativity, or power interactions in an organization.

When one is studying people, programs, organizations, or communities, the population of interest can be fairly readily determined. Constructs do not have as clear a frame of reference; neither does time.

> The problem with time sampling is that there are no concrete populations of interest, and we are anyway usually restricted to the limited time span over which a study is conducted or to the only slightly longer time span, historically speaking over

> which the literature on a topic has accumulated. For sampling operational instances of constructs, there is also no concrete target population . . . Mostly, therefore, we are forced to select on a purposive basis those particular instances of a construct that past validity studies, conventional practice, individual intuition, or consultation with critically minded persons suggest offer the closest correspondence to the construct of interest. Alternatively, we can use the same procedures to select multiple operational representations of each construct, chosen because they overlap in representing the critical theoretical components of the construct and because they differ from each other on irrelevant dimensions. This second form of sampling is called multiple operationalism, and it depends more heavily on individual judgment than does the random sampling of persons from a well-designated target population. Yet such judgments, while inevitable, are less well understood than formal sampling methods and are largely ignored by sampling experts.
> (Cook et al., 1985: 163-64)

"Operational construct" sampling simply means that one samples for study real-world examples (i.e., *operational* examples) of the constructs in which one is interested. Studying a number of such examples is called "multiple operationalism" (Webb et al., 1966).

(11) Confirming and disconfirming cases. In the early part of qualitative fieldwork the evaluator is exploring – gathering data and beginning to allow patterns to emerge. Over time the exploratory process gives way to confirmatory fieldwork. This involves testing ideas, confirming the importance and meaning of possible patterns, and checking out the viability of emergent findings with new data and additional cases. This stage of fieldwork requires considerable rigor and integrity on the part of the evaluator in looking for and sampling confirming *as well as disconfirming* cases.

Confirmatory cases are additional examples that fit already emergent patterns; these cases confirm and elaborate the findings, adding richness, depth, and credibility. Disconfirmirig cases are no less important at this point. These are the examples that don't fit. They are a source of rival interpretations as well as a way of placing boundaries around confirmed findings. They may be "exceptions that prove the rule" or exceptions that disconfirm and alter what appeared to be primary patterns.

The source of questions or ideas to be confirmed or disconfirmed maybe from stakeholders or previous scholarly literature rather than the evaluator's fieldwork. An evaluation may in part serve the purpose of confirming or disconfirming stakeholder's or scholars' preconceptions, these having been identified during early, conceptual evaluator-stakeholder design discussions or literature reviews.

Thinking aboot the challenge of finding confirming and disconfirming cases emphasizes the relationship between sampling and research conclusions. The sample determines what the evaluator will have something to say about – thus the importance of sampling carefully and thoughtfully.

(12) Opportunistic sampling. Fieldwork often involves on-the-spot decisions about sampling to take advantage of new opportunities during actual data collection. Unlike experimental designs, qualitative inquiry designs can include new sampling strategies to take advantage of unforeseen opportunities after fieldwork has begun. Being open to following wherever the data lead is a primary strength of qualitative strategies in research. This permits the sample to emerge during fieldwork.

When observing, it is not possible to capture everything. It is, therefore, necessary to make decisions about which activities to observe, which people to observe and interview, and what time periods will be selected to collect data. These decisions cannot all be made in advance. The purposeful sampling strategies discussed above often depend on some knowledge of the setting being studied. Opportunistic sampling takes advantage of whatever unfolds as it unfolds.

(13) Purposeful random sampling. The fact that a small sample size will be chosen for in-depth qualitative study does not automatically mean that the sampling strategy should not be random. For many audiences, random sampling, even of small samples, will substantially increase the credibility of the results. I recently worked with a program that annually appears before the state legislature and tells war stories' about client successes, sometimes even including a few stories about failures to provide balance. They decided they wanted to begin collecting evaluation information. Because they were striving for individualized outcomes they rejected the notion of basing the evaluation entirely on a standardized pre-post instrument. They wanted to collect case histories and do in-depth case studies of clients, but they had very limited resources and time to devote to such data collection. In effect, staff at each program site, many of whom serve 200 to 300 families a year, felt that they could only do 10 or 15 detailed, in-depth clinical case histories each year. We systematized the kind of information that would be going into the case histories at each program site and then set up a random procedure for selecting those clients whose case histories would be recorded in depth. Essentially, this program thereby systematized and randomized their collection of "war stories." While they cannot generalize to the entire client population on the basis of 10 cases from each program site, they will be able to tell legislators that the stories they are reporting were randomly selected *in advance of knowledge of how the outcomes would appear* and that the information collected was comprehensive. The credibility of systematic and randomly selected case examples is considerably greater than the personal, ad hoc selection of cases to report *after* the fact – that is, after outcomes are known.

It is critical to understand, however, that this is a purposeful random sample, not a representative random sample. *The purpose of a small random sample is credibility, not representativeness.* A small, purposeful random sample aims to reduce suspicion about why certain cases were selected for study, but such a sample still does not permit statistical generalizations.

(14) Sampling politically important cases. Evaluation is inherently and inevitably political to some extent (see Palumbo, 1987; Patton, 1986, 1987b; Turpin, 1989). A variation of the critical case sampling strategy involves selecting (or sometimes avoiding) a politically sensitive site or unit of analysis. For example, a statewide program may have a local site in the district of a state legislator who is particularly influential. By studying carefully the program in that district, evaluation data may be more likely to attract attention and get used. This does not mean that the evaluator then undertakes to make that site look either good or bad, depending on the politics of the moment. This is simply an additional sampling strategy for trying to increase the usefulness and utilization of information where resources permit the study of only a limited number of cases.

The same (broadly speaking) political perspective may inform case sampling in applied or even basic research studies. A political scientist or historian might select the Watergate or Iran-Contra scandals for study not only because of the insights they provide about the American sytem of government but because of the likely attention such a study would attract. A sociologist's study of a riot or a psychologist's study of a famous suicide would likely involve some attention during sampling to the political importance of the case.

(15) Convenience sampling. Finally, there is the strategy of sampling by convenience: doing what's fast and convenient. This is probably the most common sampling strategy – and the least desirable. Too often evaluators using qualitative methods think that, because the sample size they can study is too small to permit generalizations, it doesn't matter how cases are picked, so they might as well pick ones that are easy to access and inexpensive to study. *While convenience and cost are real considerations, they should be the last factors to be taken into account* after strategically deliberating on how to get the most in formation of greatest utility from the limited number of cases to be sampled. Purposeful, strategic sampling can yield crucial information about critical cases. *Convenience sampling is neither purposeful nor strategic.*

Information-Rich Cases

Table 5.5 summarizes the 15 purposeful sampling strategies discussed above, plus a 16th approach-combination or mixed purposeful sampling. For example, an extreme group or maximum heterogeneity approach may yield an initial potential sample size that is still larger than the study can handle. The final selection, then, may be made randomly a combination approach. Thus these approaches are not mutually exclusive. Each approach serves a somewhat different purpose. Because research and evaluations often serve multiple purposes,

Table 5.5

Sampling Strategies

Type	Purpose
A. Random probability sampling	Representativeness: Sample size a function of population size and desired confidence level.
1. simple random sample	Permits generalization from sample to the population it represents.
2. stratified random and cluster samples	Increases confidence in making generalizations to particular subgroups or areas.
B. Purposeful sampling	Selects information-rich cases for in-depth study. Size and specific cases depend on study purpose.
1. extreme or deviant case sampling	Learning from highly unusual manifestations of the phenomenon of interest, such as outstanding successes/notable failures, top of the class/dropouts, exotic events, crises.
2. intensity sampling	Information-rich cases that manifest the phenomenon intensely, but not extremely, such as good students/poor students, above average/below average.
3. maximum variation sampling – purposefully picking a wide range of variation on dimensions of interest	Documents unique or diverse variations that have emerged in adapting to different conditions. Identifies important common patterns that cut across variations.
4. homogeneous sampling	Focuses, reduces variation, simplifies analysis, facilitates group interviewing.
5. typical case sampling	Illustrates or highlights what is typical, normal, average.
6. stratified purposeful sampling	Illustrates characteristics of particular subgroups of interest; facilitates comparisons.
7. critical case sampling	Permits *logical* generalization and maximum application of information to other cases because if it's true of this one case it's likely to be true of all other cases.
8 snowball or chain sampling	Identifies cases of interest from people who know people who know people who know what cases are in formation-rich, that is, good examples for study, good interview subjects.
9. criterion sampling	Picking all cases that meet some criterion, such as all children abused in a treatment facility. Quality assurance.
10. theory-based or operational construct sampling	Finding manifestations of a theoretical construct of interest so as to elaborate and examine the construct.
11. confirming and disconfirming cases	Elaborating and deepening initial analysis, seeking exceptions, testing variation.
12. opportunistic sampling	Following new leads during fieldwork, taking advantage of the unexpected, flexibility.
13. random purposeful sampling (still small sample size)	Adds credibility to sample when potential purposeful sample is larger than one can handle. Reduces judgment within a purposeful category. (Not for generalizations or representaliveness.)
14. sampling politically important cases	Attracts attention to the study (or avoids attracting undesired attention by purposefully eliminating from the sample politically sensitive cases).
15. convenience sampling	Saves time, money, and effort: Poorest rationale; lowest credibility. Yields information-poor cases.
16. combination or mixed purposeful sampling	Triangulation, flexibility meets multiple interests and needs.

ARTICLE 12

more than one qualitative sampling strategy may be necessary. In long-term fieldwork all of these strategies may be used at some point.

These are not the only ways of sampling qualitatively. The underlying principle that is common to all these strategies is selecting information-rich cases. These are cases from which one can learn a great deal about matters of importance. They are cases worthy of in-depth study.

In the process of developing the research design, the evaluator or researcher is trying to consider and anticipate the kinds of arguments that will lend credibility to the study as well as the kinds of arguments that might be used to attack the findings. Reasons for site selections or individual case sampling need to be carefully articulated and made explicit. Moreover it is important to be open and clear about the study's limitations, including how any particular purposeful sampling strategy may lead to distortion in the findings – that is, to anticipate criticisms that will be made of a particular sampling strategy.

Having weighed the evidence and considered the alternatives, evaluators and primary stakeholders make their sampling decisions, sometimes painfully, but always with the recognition that there are no perfect designs. The sampling strategy must be selected to fit the purpose of the study, the resources available, the questions being asked, and the constraints being faced. This holds true for sampling strategy as well as sample size.

SAMPLE SIZE

Qualitative inquiry is rife with ambiguities. There are purposeful strategies instead of methodological rules. There are inquiry approaches instead of statistical formulas. Qualitative inquiry seems to work best for people with a high tolerance for ambiguity. (And we're still only discussing design. It gets worse when we get to analysis.)
Nowhere is this ambiguity clearer than in the matter of sample size.

I get letters. I get calls. "Is 10 a large enough sample to achieve maximum variation?"

"I started out to interview 20 people for 2 hours each, but I've lost 2 people. Is 18 large enough, or do I have to find 2 more?"

"I want to study just one organization, but interview 20 people in the organization. Is my sample size 1 or 20 or both?"

My universal, certain, and confident reply to these questions is this: "*it depends.*"

There are no rules for sample size in qualitative inquiry. Sample size depends on what you want to know, the purpose of the inquiry, what's at stake, what will be useful, what will have credibility, and what can be done with available time and resources.

Earlier in this chapter, I discussed the trade-off between breadth and depth. With the same fixed resources and limited time, a researcher could study a

specific set of experiences for a larger number of people (seeking breadth) or a more open range of experiences for a smaller number of people (seeking depth). In-depth information from a small number of people can be very valuable, especially if the cases are information-rich. Less depth from a large number of people can be especially helpful in exploring a phenomenon and trying to document diversity or understand variation. I repeat, the size of the sample depends on what you want to find out, why you want to find it out, how the findings will be used, and what resources (including time) you have for the study

To understand the problem of small samples in qualitative inquiry, it's necessary to place these small samples in the context of probability sampling. A qualitative inquiry sample only seems small in comparison with the sample size needed for representativeness when the purpose is generalizing from a sample to the population of which it is a part. Suppose there are 100 people in a program to be evaluated. It would be necessary to randomly sample 80 of those people (80%) to make a generalization at the 95% confidence level. If there are 500 people in the program, 217 people must be sampled (43%) for the same level of confidence. If there are 1,000 people, 278 people must be sampled (28%); and if there are 5,000 people in the population of interest, 357 must be sampled (7%) to achieve a 95% confidence level in the generalization of findings. At the other extreme, if there are only 50 people in the program, 44 must be randomly sampled (88%) to achieve a 95% level of confidence. (See Fitzgibbon and Morris, 1987: 163, for a table on determining sample size from a given population.)

The logic of purposeful sampling is quite different from the logic of probability sampling. The problem is, however, that the utility and credibility of small purposeful samples are often judged on the basis of the logic, purpose, and recommended sample sizes of probability sampling. What should happen is that purposeful samples be judged on the basis of the purpose and rationale of each study and the sampling strategy used to achieve the study's purpose. The sample, like all other aspects of qualitative inquiry, must be judged in context the same principle that undergirds analysis and presentation of qualitative data. Random probability samples cannot accomplish what in-depth, purposeful samples accomplish, and vice versa.

Piaget contributed a major breakthrough to our understanding of how children think by observing his own two children at length and in great depth. Freud established the field of psychoanalysis based on fewer than ten client cases. Bandler and Crinder (1975a, 1975b) founded neurolinguistic programming (NLP) by studying three renowned and highly effective therapists: Milton Erickson, Fritz Perls, and Virginia Satir. Peters and Waterman (1982) formulated their widely followed eight principles for organizational excellence by studying 62 companies, a very small sample of the thousands of companies one might study.

The validity, meaningfulness, and insights generated from qualitative inquiry have more to do with the information-richness of the cases selected and the observational/analytical capabilities of the researcher than with sample size.

This issue of sample size is a lot like the problem students have when they are assigned an essay to write.

Student: "How long does the paper have to be?"
Instructor: "Long enough to cover the assignment."
Student: "But how many pages?"
Instructor: "Enough pages to do justice to the subject – no more, no less."

Lincoln and Guba (1985: 202) recommend sample selection

to the point of redundancy . . . In purposeful sampling the size of the sample is determined by informational considerations. If the purpose is to maximize information, the sampling is terminated when no new information is forthcoming from new sampled units; thus *redundancy* is the primary criterion. (emphasis in the original)

This strategy leaves the question of sample size open.

There remains, however, the practical problems of how to negotiate an evaluation budget or how to get a dissertation committee to approve a design if you don't have some idea of sample size. Sampling to the point of redundancy is an ideal, one that works best for basic research, unlimited time lines, and unconstrained resources.

The solution is judgment and negotiation. I recommended that qualitative sampling designs specify minimum samples based on expected reasonable coverage of the phenomenon given the purpose of the study and stakeholder interests. One may add to the sample as fieldwork unfolds. One may change the sample if information emerges that indicates the value of a change. The design should be understood to be flexible and emergent. Yet, at the beginning, for planning and budgetary purposes, one specifies a minimum expected sample size and builds a rationale for that minimum, as well as criteria that would alert the researcher to inadequacies in the original sampling approach and/or size.

In the end, sample size adequacy, like all aspects of research, is subject to peer review, consensual validation, and judgment. What is crucial is that the sampling procedures and decisions be fully described, explained, and justified so that information users and peer reviewers have the appropriate context for judging the sample. The researcher or evaluator is absolutely obligated to discuss how the sample affected the findings, the strengths and weaknesses of the sampling procedures, and any other design decisions that are relevant for interpreting and understanding the reported results. Exercising care not to overgeneralize from

purposeful samples, while maximizing to the full the advantages of in-depth, purposeful sampling, will do much to alleviate concerns about small sample size.

METHODOLOGICAL MIXES

A study may employ more than one sampling strategy. It may also include multiple types of data. The chapters on interviewing, observation, and analysis will include information that will help in making design decisions. Before turning to those chapters, however I want to briefly discuss the value of using multiple methods in research and evaluation.

Triangulation

One important way to strengthen a study design is through triangulation, or the combination of methodologies in the study of the same phenomena or programs. This can mean using several kinds of methods or data, including using both quantitative and qualitative approaches. Denzin (1978b) has identified four basic types of triangulation: (1) *data triangulation* – the use of a variety of data sources in a study; (2) *investigator triangulation* – the use of several different researchers or evaluators; (3) *theory triangulation* – the use of multiple perspectives to interpret a single set of data; and (4) *methodological triangulation* – the use of multiple methods to study a single problem or program.

The term *triangulation* is taken from land surveying. Knowing a single landmark only locates you somewhere along a line in a direction from the landmark, whereas with two landmarks you can take bearings in two directions and locate yourself at their intersection (Fielding and Fielding, 1986: 23). The term *triangulation* also works metaphorically to call to mind the world's strongest geometric shape – the triangle (e.g., the form used to construct geodesic domes à la Buckminster Fuller). The logic of triangulation is based on the premise that

no single method ever adequately solves the problem of rival causal factors. . . . Because each method reveals different aspects of empirical reality, multiple methods of observations must be employed. This is termed triangulation. I now offer as a final methodological rule the principle that multiple methods should be used in every investigation. (Denzin, 1978b: 28)

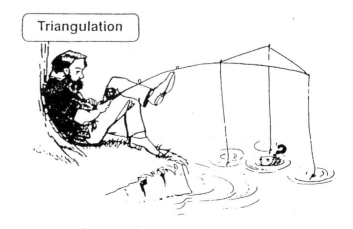

Triangulation

Triangulation is ideal. It can also be very expensive. An evaluation's limited budget, short time frame, and political constraints will affect the amount of triangulation that is practical. Certainly, one important strategy for conducting evaluation research is to employ multiple methods, measures, researchers, and perspectives – but to do so reasonably and practically. Combinations of interviewing, observation, and document analysis are expected in much social science fieldwork. Other studies may rely only on interviews or observations. Studies that use only one method are more vulnerable to errors linked to that particular method (e.g., loaded interview questions, biased or untrue responses) than studies that use multiple methods in which different types of data provide cross-data validity checks.

It is possible to achieve triangulation within a qualitative inquiry strategy by combining different kinds of qualitative methods, mixing purposeful samples, and including multiple perspectives. It is also possible to cut across inquiry approaches and achieve triangulation by combining qualitative and quantitative methods, a strategy discussed and illustrated in the next section. For an excellent review of the strengths and weaknesses of many different data collection techniques, see Marshall and Rossman (1989:102-5).

Mixing Data, Design, and Analysis Approaches

Triangulation can include borrowing and combining parts from pure methodological approaches, thus creating mixed methodological strategies. To accomplish this it is necessary to separate the measurement, design, and analysis components of the hypothetico-deductive (quantitative/experimental) and holistic-inductive (qualitative/naturalistic) paradigms discussed in Chapter 2. The ideal-typical qualitative methods strategy is made up of three parts: (1) qualitative data, (2) a holistic-inductive design of naturalistic inquiry, and (3) content or case analysis. In the traditional hypothetico-deductive approach to research, the ideal study would include (a) quantitative data from (b) experimental (or quasi-experimental) designs and (c) statistical analysis.

A variety of mixes are possible – mixes of measurement, design, and analysis. At this point these mixes may seem abstract. In order to make the choices available more concrete, and to illustrate the creative possibilities that can emerge out of flexible approaches to research design, it may be helpful to examine alternative mixes of measurement, design, and analysis for a single program evaluation. The examples that follow have been constructed under the artificial constraint that only one kind of measurement, design, and analysis could be used in each case. In practice, of course, the possible mixes are much more varied, because any given study could include several measurement approaches, varying design approaches, and varying different analytical approaches to achieve triangulation.

The Case of Operation Reach-Out: Variations in Program Evaluation Design

With funds provided by United Way, local foundations, and state government, a comprehensive program is established in a major city to serve high school age students who are at high risk educationally (poor grades, poor attendance, poor attitudes toward school), highly vulnerable in terms of their health (poor nutrition, sedentary life-style, high drug use), and likely candidates for contact with the criminal justice system (histories of juvenile delinquency, poor employment prospects, and alienation from dominant societal values). The program consists of experiential education internships through which these high risk students get individual tutoring in basic skills, part-time job placements that permit them to earn income while gaining work exposure, and participation in peer group discussions aimed at changing health values, establishing a positive peer culture, and increasing social integration. The mandate for the program includes a requirement that the program be evaluated. Several evaluation approaches are possible. Each approach that follows illustrates a different strategy.

Pure Hypothetical-Deductive Approach to Evaluation: Experimental Design, Quantitative Data, and Statistical Analysis

The evaluator determines that the program does not have sufficient resources to include all of the youth in the target population. Therefore, a pool of eligible youth is established with admission into the program on a random basis and the remaining group receiving no treatment intervention. Before the program begins and one year later, all youth, both those in the program and those in the control group, are administered standardized instruments measuring school achievement, self-esteem, anomie, alienation, and locus of control. Rates of school attendance, sickness, drug use, and delinquency are obtained for each group. When all data have been collected at the end of the year, comparisons between the control and experimental groups are made using inferential statistics.

Pure Qualitative Strategy: Naturalistic Inquiry, Qualitative Data, and Content Analysis

Procedures for recruiting and selecting participants for the program are determined entirely by the staff. The evaluator finds a convenient time to conduct an in-depth interview with participants as soon as they are admitted into the program. These in-depth interviews ask students to describe what school is like for them, what they do in school, how they typically spend their time, what their family life is like, how they approach academic tasks, their views about health, and their behaviors/attitudes with regard to delinquent and criminal activity In brief, participants are asked to describe themselves and their social world. The evaluator finds out from program staff when the program activities will be taking place and observes those activities, collecting detailed data about what happens during those activities: participant behaviors, participant conversations, staff behaviors, staff-paticipant interactions, and related phenomena. During the course of the program the evaluator finds convenient opportunities for conducting additional in-depth interviews with participants to find out how they view the program, what kinds of experiences they are having, and what they are doing. Near the end of the program, in-depth interviews are conducted with the participants to find out what behaviors have changed, how they view things, and what their expectations are for the future. In-depth interviews are also conducted with program staff. These data are content analyzed to identify the patterns of experience participants bring to the program, what patterns characterize their participation in the program, and what patterns of change are reported by and observed in the participants.

Mixed Form: Experimental Design, Qualitative Data, and Content Analysis

As in the pure experimental form, potential participants are randomly assigned to treatment and control groups. In-depth interviews are conducted with all youth, both those in the treatment group and those in the control group, before the program begins. The focus of those interviews is similar to that in the pure qualitative approach. Interviews are conducted again at the end of the program. Content analysis is perfonned separately on the data from the control group and the experimental group. The patterns found in the control group and the experimental group are then compared and contrasted.

Mixed Form: Experimental Design, Qualitative Data, and Statistical Analysis

Participants are randomly assigned to treatment and control groups, and in-depth interviews are conducted both before the program and at the end of the program. These interview data, in raw form, are then given to a panel of judges who rate each interview along several outcome dimensions operationalized as a ten-point scale. For both the "pre" interview and the "post" interview, the judges assign ratings on such dimensions as likelihood of success in school (low = 1 high = 10), likelihood of committing criminal offenses (low = 1, high = 10), commitment to education, commitment to engaging in productive work, self-esteem, and manifestation of desired nutritional and health habits. Inferential statistics are then used to compare these two groups. Judges make the ratings without knowledge of which participants were in which group. Outcomes on the rated scales are also statistically related to background characteristics of participants.

Mixed Form: Naturalistic Inquiry Qualitative Data, Statistical Analysis

As in the pure qualitative form, students are selected for the program on the basis of whatever criteria staff choose to apply. In-depth interviews are conducted with all students before the program and at the end of the program. These data are then submitted to a panel of judges, who rate them on a series of dimensions similar to those listed in the previous example. Change scores are computed for each individual, and changes arc statistically related to background characteristics of the students to determine in a regression format which characteristics of students are likely to predict success in the program. In addition, observations of program activities are rated on a set of scales developed to quantify the climate attributes of activities: for example, the extent to which the activity involved active or passive participation, the extent to which student-teacher interaction was high or low, the extent to which interactions were formal or info..rinal, and the extent to which participants had input into program activities. Ratings of activities based on qualitative descriptions are then aggregated to provide an overview of the treatment environment of the program.

Mixed Form: Naturalistic Inquiry, Quantitative Data, Statistical Analysis

Students are selected for the program according to staff criteria. The evaluator enters the program setting without any predetermined categories of analysis or presuppositions about important variables or variable relationships. The evaluator observes important activities and events in the program, looking for the types of behaviors and interactions that will emerge. For each new type of behavior or interaction, the evaluator creates a category and then uses a time and space sampling design to count the frequency with which those categories of behavior and interaction are exhibited. The frequency of the manifestation of observed behaviors and interactions are then statistically related to such characteristics as group size, duration of the activity, staff-student ratios, and social/physical density.

Pure Versus Mixed Strategies

Triangulation is a powerful solution to the problem of relying too much on any single data source or method, thereby undermining the validity and credibility of findings because of the weaknesses of any single method. Using triangulation is recognition that the researcher needs to be open to more than one way of looking at things. A corollary to this insight is that purity of method is less important than dedication to relevant and useful information. I shall return to the ways in which triangulation can enhance data quality and the credibility of findings in Chapter 9. Having presented some of the ways in which a practical and utilitarian design for evaluation may involve departures from methodological purity, it is worth considering the case for maintaining the integrity and purity of each methodological approach, model, or paradigm.

There are strong arguments for maintaining the integrity of a pure qualitative methods approach in evaluation. The themes of qualitative methods described

ARTICLE 12

in the second chapter do fit together into a cohesive approach. The openness and personal involvement of naturalistic inquiry mesh well with the openness and depth of qualitative data. Genuine openness flows naturally from an inductive approach to analysis, particularly an analysis grounded in the immediacy of direct fieldwork and sensitized to the desirability of holistic understanding of unique human settings.

Likewise, there is an internal consistency and logic to quantitative experimental designs, which test deductive hypotheses derived from theoretical premises. These premises identify the key variables to consider in measuring, controlling, and analyzing important program treatments and outcomes. The rules and procedures of the quantitative-experimental paradigm are aimed at producing internally valid, reliable, replicable, and generalizable findings.

Guba and Lincoln (1988) have argued that the internal consistency and logic of each approach, or paradigm, mitigates against methodological mixing of different inquiry modes and data-collection strategies. Their cautions are not to be dismissed lightly. Mixing parts of different approaches is a matter of philosophical and methodological controversy. Yet, the practical mandate in evaluation (Patton, 1981) to gather the most relevant possible information for evaluation users outweighs concerns about methodological purity based on epistemological and philosophical arguments. The intellectual mandate to be open to what the world has to offer surely includes methodological openness. In practice it is altogether possible, as we have seen, to combine approaches, and to do so creatively (Patton, l987a).

Advocates of methodological purity argue that a single evaluator cannot be both deductive and inductive at the same time; one cannot be testing predetermined hypotheses and still remain open to whatever emerges from open-ended, phenomenological observation. Yet, in practice, human reasoning is sufficiently complex and flexible that it is possible to research predetermined questions and test hypotheses about certain aspects of a program while being quite open and naturalistic in pursuing other aspects of a program. In principle, this is not greatly different from a questionnaire that includes both fixed alternative and open-ended questions. The extent to which a qualitative approach is inductive or deductive varies along a continuum. As evaluation fieldwork begins, the evaluator may be open to whatever emerges from the data, a discovery or inductive approach. Then, as the inquiry reveals patterns and major dimensions of interest, the evaluator will begin to focus on verifying and elucidating what appears to be emerging – a more deductive approach to data collection and analysis.

The extent to which a study is "naturalistic" in design is also a matter of degree. This applies particularly with regard to the extent to which the evaluator places conceptual constraints on or makes presuppositions about the program. In practice, the naturalistic approach may often involve moving back and forth between inductive, open-ended, and phenomenological encounters with

programs to more hypothetical-deductive attempts to verify "hypotheses" or solidify ideas that emerged from those more open-ended experiences, sometimes even manipulating something to to see what happens. These and other variations on qualitative inquiry were explored at the end of Chapter 2.

These examples of variations in qualitative approaches are somewhat like the differences between experimental and quasi-experimental designs. Pure experiments are the ideal; quasi-experimental designs often represent what is possible and practical. Likewise, full participant observation over an extended period of time is the qualitative ideal. In practice, there are many acceptable and meaningful variations in using qualitative methods.

This spirit of adaptability and creativity in designing evaluations is aimed at being responsive to real-world conditions and meeting stakeholder information needs. It is in this spirit that I conclude this chapter with a final discussion of making methods decisions.

Making Decisions About Research Methods

The examples just listed provide only a few illustrations of possible research strategies. Figure 5.1 summarizes these six possibilities. It is also possible to combine strategies, although certain designs pose constraints that exclude other possibilities. It is not possible, for example, to create an experimental situation with treatment and control groups while at the same time studying the natural evolution of a program, including the natural development by program staff of criteria for selection into the program.

The examples also illustrate another limitation on mixing methods. It is possible to convert detailed, qualitative descriptions into quantitative scales for purposes of statistical analysis. It is not possible, however, to work the other way around and convert purely quantitative measures into detailed, qualitative descriptions.

Which research design is best? Which strategy will provide the most useful information to decision makers? There is no simple, immediate, and universal answer to that question. The answer in each case will depend on what intended users want to know, the purpose of the study, the funds available, the political context, and the interests/abilities/biases of the researchers. Table 5.6

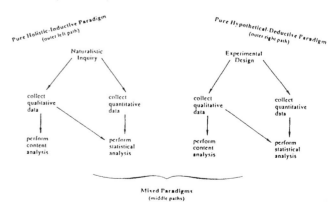

Figure 5.1. Measurement, Design, and Analysis: Pure and Mixed Combinations

Table 5.6

Design Issues and Options

Issues	Sample Options and Considerations
1. What is the primary purpose of the study?	Basic research, applied research, summative evaluation, formative evaluation, action research
2. What is the focus of study?	Breadth versus depth trade-offs
3. What are the units of analysis?	Individuals, groups, program components, whole programs, organizations, communities, critical incidents, time periods, and so on
4. What will be the sampling strategy or strategies?	Purposeful sampling, probability sampling; variations in sample size from a single case study to a generalizable sample
5. What types of data will be collected?	Qualitative, quantitative, or both
6. What controls will be exercised?	Naturalistic inquiry, experimental design, quasi-experimental options
7. What analytical approach or approaches will be used?	Inductive, deductive
	Content analysis, statistical analysis, combinations
8. How will validity of and confidence in the findings be addressed?	Triangulation options, multiple data sources, multiple methods, multiple perspectives, and multiple investigators
9. Time Issues: When will the study occur? How will the study sequenced or phased?	Long-term fieldwork, rapid reconnaissance, exploratory phase to confirmatory phase, fixed times versus open time lines
10. How will logistics and practicalities be handled?	Gaining entry to the setting, access to people and records, contracts, training, endurance, and so on
11. How will ethical issues and matters of confidentiality be handled?	Informed consent, protection of human subjects, reactivity, presentation of self, and so on
12. What resources will be available? What will the study cost?	Personnel, supplies, data collection, materials, analysis time and costs, reporting/publishing costs

ARTICLE 12

summarizes the issues discussed in this chapter that are typically necessary to address in designing a study.

In qualitative inquiry the problem of design poses a "paradox." The term design suggests a very specific blueprint, but "design in the naturalistic sense . . . means planning for certain broad contingencies without, however, indicating exactly what will be done in relation to each" (Lincoln and Guba, 1985: 226). A qualitative design needs to remain sufficiently open and flexible to permit exploration of whatever the phenomenon under study offers for inquiry. Qualitative designs continue to be emergent even after data collection begins. The degree of flexibility and openness is, however also a matter of great variation among designs.

What is certain is that different methods produce quite different information. The challenge is to find out which information is most needed and most useful in a given situation, and then to employ those methods best suited to producing the needed information. Martin Trow (1970) points out (quite nicely, I think) the difference between arguments about which methods are most appropriate for studying a particular problem as opposed to arguments about the intrinsic and universal superiority of one method over another.

> Every cobbler thinks leather is the only thing. Most social scientists, including the present writer have their favorite research methods with which they are familiar and have some skill in using. And I suspect we mostly choose to investigate problems that seem vulnerable to attack through these methods. But we should at least try to be less parochial than cobblers. Let us be done with the arguments of participant observation *versus* interviewing – as we have largely dispensed with the arguments for psychology *versus* sociology – and get on with the business of attacking our problems with the widest array of conceptual and methodological tools that we possess and they demand. This does not preclude discussion and debate regarding the relative usefulness of different methods for the study of specific problems or types of problems. But that is very different from the assertion of the general and inherent superiority of one method over another on the basis of some intrinsic qualities it presumably possesses. (Trow, 1970: 149, emphasis in the original)

CHOICES

The second chapter suggested that evaluation research should be built on the foundation of a "paradigm of choices" rather than become the handmaiden of any single, narrow disciplinary or methodological paradigm. But be careful, the Sufis would warn us, for the exercise of real choice can be elusive. Trow admonishes us to "at least try to be less parochial than cobblers." The evaluation sage, Halcolm, might suggest that all too often the methods choices made by evaluators are like the bear's decision to like honey.

> One day, in a sudden impulse of generosity, a bear decided to enlighten the other animals in the forest about the marvelous properties of honey. The bear assembled all the other animals together for his momentous announcement.
>
> "I have studied the matter at great length," began the bear "and I have decided that honey is the best of all foods. Therefore, I have chosen to like honey. I am going to describe to you the perfect qualities of honey which, due to your past prejudices and lack of experience, you have ignored. Then you will be able to make the same rational decision that I have made.
>
> "Honey comes conveniently packaged in beautifully shaped prisms of the most delicate texture. It's ready to eat, slides down the throat ever so easily, is a highly nutritious source of energy, digests smoothly, and leaves a lingering taste of sweetness on the palate that provides pleasure for hours. Honey is readily available and requires no special labor to produce since bees do all the work. Its pleasing aroma, light weight, resistance to spoilage, and uniformly high quality make it a food beyond compare. It comes ready to consume – no peeling, no killing, no tearing open – and there's no waste What's more, it has so many uses; it can be eaten alone or added as an improvement to any other food.
>
> "I could go on and on, but suffice it to say that I have studied the situation quite objectively and at great length. A fair and rational analysis leads to only one conclusion. Honey is the supreme food and any reasonable animal will undoubtedly make the same conscious decision I have made. I have chosen to like honey."

This chapter was first published by Routledge and is reproduced by permission of Routledge

DEVELOPMENTS IN QUALITATIVE DATA ANALYSIS: AN INTRODUCTION

Alan Bryman and Robert G. Burgess

Analysing Qualitative Data, London: Routledge, 1994

The last decade has witnessed several shifts in emphasis among teachers and researchers when dealing with research methodology. First, method has given way to a discussion of methodology. Second, the pre-eminence and predominance of quantitative methodology has been replaced by an emphasis upon qualitative methodology in British sociology. Third, stages of social investigation have been replaced with the idea of research as a social process which requires careful scrutiny. Each of these developments has had an impact upon the other and in turn holds implications for the way in which the analysis of qualitative data is conducted and discussed. On this basis, it is important to examine each of these trends before turning to a detailed examination of a range of approaches to qualitative data analysis that is presented in the essays in this volume.

Despite discussions of the difficulties associated with conducting social research and the importance of adapting the principles of social investigation in the conduct of particular studies, it is apparent that the teaching of research methodology has until the recent past placed little emphasis either upon research practice or upon methodology as such. The course outlines (Peel 1968, Wakeford 1979) that have been collected from those engaged in teaching such courses to undergraduates in sociology demonstrate that there has been a strong emphasis upon the teaching of techniques. Indeed, this is also demonstrated in the most popular texts used by teachers (Marsh 1979). According to these outlines the three most widely cited methods texts that were used on undergraduate methods courses were Aaron Cicourel's *Method and Measurement in Sociology* (1964), Moser and Kalton's *Survey Methods in Social Investigation* (1971), and Oppenheim's *Questionnaire Design and Attitude Measurement* (1966). As Bulmer and Burgess (1981) remarked, Cicourel may provide a critical edge to methods teaching, but may also lead students away from empirical investigation. Meanwhile, the volumes by Moser and Kalton and Oppenheim give a focus to 'methods' which emphasize techniques: sampling, questionnaire design, interviewing and so on. Yet, the volume by Moser and Kalton gives little status to the diverse range of approaches covered by the term 'qualitative methods', which are briefly summarized in one chapter.

This approach to 'methods' was the subject of considerable revision in the 1980s, which witnessed the publication of a range of volumes focusing upon qualitative research. These included general texts (Burgess 1984a, Hammersley and Atkinson 1983) as well as more specialist volumes that took up aspects of qualitative research such as policy (Finch 1986), writing (Atkinson 1990), ethics (Burgess 1989), and reading and evaluating texts (Hammersley 1991). While many of these books focused upon major elements of research, there was little emphasis given to data analysis and only Miles and Huberman (1984) devoted a whole volume to this topic; in it principles of data analysis were discussed, although not in relation to research studies that had been conducted recently. However, one important aspect of research that was revealed in these texts was a shift from 'methods' and 'stages' of social research to a discussion of methodology in terms of a research process.

These trends in research and writing were also reflected in texts recommended on undergraduate courses concerned with social research. In the academic year 1990-1, Jon Gubbay conducted a project on the teaching of undergraduate sociology which included a special study of research methods teaching. By examining lists of recommended texts on sixty-eight 'research methods' courses, he found that the 'top seven' volumes included three books concerned with qualitative research: Burgess's *In the Field* (1984a), Hammersley and Atkinson's *Ethnography: Principles in Practice* (1983) and Burgess's *Field Research: a Sourcebook and Field Manual* (1982). However, it is interesting to note that the most frequently used volume was De Vaus's book on survey research (1991), alongside a wide range of volumes on quantitative and qualitative methodology.[1] Such a range of volumes indicated an emphasis on the practice of social research and a welcome attempt to teach quantitative and qualitative research.

Many of the volumes on qualitative research emphasized the research process and demonstrated that qualitative research cannot be reduced to particular techniques nor to set stages, but rather that a dynamic process is involved which links together problems, theories and methods. Here, the focus is upon the links between research design, research strategy and research techniques as well as the relationship between aspects of research design, data collection and data analysis. The importance of this approach to social research had been well summarized by Bechhofer when he stated:

The research process, then, is not a clear cut sequence of procedures following a neat pattern, but a messy interaction between the conceptual and empirical world, deduction and induction occurring at the same time. (1974: 73)

Here, the difficulties involved in doing research and writing about it are vividly portrayed through the use of the word 'messy'. Indeed, research seldom involves the use of a straightforward set of procedures. Instead, the researcher has to move backwards and forwards between different sequences in the research process. For example, in designing a project, consideration needs to be given to the end-point and the concepts and theories that will be used in data analysis. Similarly, in terms of data collection, reference has to be made to the comparisons and contrasts that may be uncovered during a project. On this basis, there is not a sharp divide between different aspects of the research process in practice. Accordingly, while the contributors to this volume seek to examine critically the way in which qualitative data analysis is handled in practice, it is evident that they need to move between other aspects of the research process and qualitative data analysis, while keeping the latter as the central theme. However, before turning to some accounts of this process we need to look at some of the procedures that are advocated by those methodologists who have chosen to write about this aspect of doing research.

QUALITATIVE TEXTS

General texts on research methods have ignored qualitative data analysis despite allocating space to data collection (Frankfort-Nachmias and Nachmias 1992, Kidder and Judd 1986). Sometimes the analysis of qualitative data is only briefly covered (Babbie 1979) through 'coding' and the generation of theory from data.

It is not surprising that in texts concerned primarily with qualitative research, data analysis has been allocated fairly detailed treatments. As with the general texts, there is a tendency for gaining access, data collection strategies and fieldwork relationships to make up the bulk of the discussion before the move on to analysis (Bogdan and Biklen 1982, Bogdan and Taylor 1975, Burgess 1984a, Hammersley and Atkinson 1983, Goetz and LeCompte 1984, Lofland 1974 and Whyte 1984). Typically, these treatments discuss the major strategies for analyzing qualitative data, frequently using examples from the writers' own or others' research. In recent years, some books which focus more or less exclusively on qualitative data analysis have emerged. One of the best known is Miles and Huberman (1984), which offers a distinctive approach. Strauss (1987) and Strauss and Corbin (1990) provide detailed elaborations of grounded theory, while Tesch (1990) and Fielding and Lee (1991) pay a great deal of attention to analysis in the context of the development of computer software, which is increasingly being used by researchers. Two

main approaches to qualitative data analysis can be found in texts: first, a discussion of the main general frameworks; second, provision of the main emphases of qualitative data analysis. These two approaches can be described as 'general strategies' and 'general processes', to which we now turn.

GENERAL STRATEGIES

The general strategies approach can be found in such texts as Bryman (1988), Burgess (1984a) and Hammersley (1989, 1992), as well as Bulmer's (1979) examination of concept generation during the analysis of qualitative data. The usual approach involves an articulation of two of the best known general strategies: analytic induction and grounded theory.

Analytic induction is closely associated with studies of social problems, though it has more general applicability. Its main elements have been outlined by Robinson (1951) and comprise a sequence of steps. The researcher begins with a rough definition of a problem or issue (e.g. drug addiction). Appropriate cases are examined and a possible explanation of the problem is formulated and the investigator then examines further appropriate cases to establish how well the data collected fit the hypothetical explanation. If there is a lack of fit, the hypothesis is likely to need reformulation and further research is conducted. There then follows an iterative interplay between data collection and revision of the hypothesis as research reveals cases that do not fit with each reformulated hypothesis. Indeed, the original problem itself may be redefined in the process. The sequence continues until cases that are inconsistent with what ends up as the last reformulated hypothesis do not appear. Analytic induction is extremely demanding in that the appearance of a single case that is inconsistent with a hypothesis (or a reformulated one) necessitates further revision of the hypothesis and a return to the field. However, there are very few instances of the use of analytic induction and it is striking that writers such as Bryman (1988) and Hammersley (1989) employ old studies – Lindesmith (1947) and Cressey (1950) respectively as illustrations. It may be that the extremely stringent requirements implied by analytic induction have been responsible for its relatively infrequent use.

Grounded theory bears certain similarities to analytic induction in respect of the meshing of theorizing and data collection. Detailed presentations of the approach can be found in Glaser and Strauss (1967), Strauss (1987) and Strauss and Corbin (1990), but Turner 1981 (see also Martin and Turner 1986) has provided an especially helpful account of its main steps, which collectively are concerned with 'the discovery of theory from data' (Glaser and Strauss 1967: 1). After some data collection and reflection in relation to a general issue of concern, the researcher generates 'categories' which fit the data. Further research is undertaken until the categories are 'saturated', that is, the researcher feels assured about their meaning and importance. The researcher then attempts to formulate more general (and possibly more abstract) expressions of these categories, which will then be capable of embracing a wider range of objects. This stage may spur the researcher to further theoretical reflection and in particular he or she should by now be concerned with the interconnections among the categories involved and their generality. Hypotheses about links between categories will need to be formulated and tested in the field. Links with other theoretical schemes are then explored and as further revisions of hypotheses are carried out, as a result of both data collection and theoretical reflection, the emerging theory is tested once again in the field.

Coding represents a key step in the process. It has been described by Charmaz (1983) as 'simply the process of categorizing and sorting data' (p. 111), while 'codes' are described as serving to 'summarize, synthesize, and sort many observations made out of the data' (p. 112). As such, coding provides the link between data and the conceptualization. At first, the coding will be 'open coding' (Strauss 1987), or 'initial coding' as it was referred to in earlier writings on grounded theory (Charmaz 1983, Glaser 1978): 'the process of breaking down, examining, comparing, conceptualizing, and categorizing data' (Strauss and Corbin 1990: 61); coding here represents the gradual building up of categories out of the data. Later, 'axial coding' will be employed. This involves 'a set of procedures whereby data are put back together in new ways after open coding, by making connections between categories' (1990: 96). It should be noted that, as Richards and Richards (1991) observe, the term 'coding' is widely used in qualitative analysis but is applied in more than one way: to the task of fitting data and concepts together in such a way that conceptualization is under constant revision (as in grounded theory); to a process that is more or less identical to the coding of open-ended questions in survey research, where the aim is to quantify different categories of a variable.[2] Another key element in grounded theory is 'memo writing', whereby the analyst is constantly writing memos, perhaps relating to codes or to connections between emerging concepts, which elaborate the data and which represent the first step in the emergence of theory.

Grounded theory has been widely cited and writers of computer software for qualitative analysis often claim that it influenced their construction of the programs or that the programs were designed with doing grounded theory in mind (see Seidel and Clark 1984: 112, and Richards and Richards, this volume). The part played by grounded theory can be discerned very clearly in the following account by Sutton of how he analyzed his data on 'dying' organizations to produce a 'process model of organisational death':

> The method of data analysis used here draws on recommendations by Glaser and Strauss (1967) and Miles and Huberman (1984). The method entailed continuous comparison of data and model throughout the research project. I began the research by developing a rough working framework based on the existing literature, conversations with colleagues, and pilot interviews. I travelled back and forth between the emerging model and evidence throughout the data gathering and writing. In doing so, some elements suggested by the literature and prior intuitions could be grounded in evidence, while others could not. Other elements proposed at the outset or suggested by a subset of cases were retained but were modified considerably to conform to the evidence.   (1987: 547)

However, in general there are relatively few genuine cases of grounded theory using the approach that is specified above. Very often, the term is employed in research publications to denote an approach to data analysis in which theory has emerged from the data. Rarely is there a genuine interweaving of data collection and theorizing of the kind advocated by Glaser and Strauss. Even the example of Sutton's description of his analytical procedures seems to imply that a model emerged at a much earlier stage (in terms of the amount of data collected prior to its specification) than the grounded theory approach would seem to suggest. As a result, grounded theory is probably given lip-service to a greater degree than is appreciated (Bryman 1988: 54-5). Richards and Richards make a similar point when they observe that grounded theory 'is widely adopted as an approving bumper sticker in qualitative studies' (1991: 43). Moreover, the precise process whereby a grounded theory analysis was undertaken is often imprecise.

A further strategy that has been identified by Williams (1976) and Hammersley (1989) is the *pattern model*, which does not separate explanation from description. According to this model,

> the activity of describing the relation between one action and others in a context is equivalent to interpreting or explaining the meaning of that action. Describing its place and its relation to other parts is therefore to explain it.
> (Williams 1976: 128)

However, this model operates at a higher level of generality than analytic induction and grounded theory and provides relatively few guide-lines when confronted with data.

Tesch (1991) has also identified different approaches to analysis. First are approaches based on language: discourse analysis, symbolic interactionism and ethnomethodology, in which the focus is on how language is employed. Second, there is a 'descriptive or interpretive approach', which seeks to establish a coherent and inclusive account of a culture from the point of view of those being researched. Classic ethnography and life history studies fall into this type. Finally, there are 'theory-building' approaches, as in grounded theory and in Miles and Huberman (1984), in which the generation of theory is a primary goal. The chief problem with this delineation is that it does not address the process of analysis. Also, the distinctions are not without difficulties. Tesch notes that symbolic interactionists, while being included primarily in the first category, are also concerned to build theory. It is also questionable whether the first two categories are quite as unconcerned with theory-building as the distinction implies.

GENERAL PROCESSES

The generation of concepts is one of the most frequently mentioned aspects of qualitative data analysis in the texts that have been reviewed. Hammersley and Atkinson (1983) recommended immersing oneself in the data and then searching out patterns, identifying possibly surprising phenomena, and being sensitive to inconsistencies, such as divergent views offered by different groups of individuals. They recognize that sometimes the researcher will end up generating new concepts, but on other occasions will be relating his or her observations to pre-existing notions (see Lofland 1971). Initially, the concepts may not be clearly defined and will require elaboration. As clues to the generation of new concepts, Woods (1986: 133-4) recommends being sensitive to repetitions of incidents or words, irregularities, unusual occurrences and how people say things (for example, if accompanied by droll laughter, embarrassment, anger). He shows how his notion of teachers' survival strategies was built up from such evidence as a series of well-prepared eighty-minute science classes to which the pupils were paying next to no attention or from utterly chaotic lessons which teachers regarded as having gone down well. Miles and Huberman (1984: 60) observe that there will be a close connection between coding and the generation of concepts, regardless of whether the latter are pre-specified (and later revised) or emergent. However, for most practitioners codes are the building blocks for emergent rather than pre-specified concepts.

Hammersley and Atkinson (1983), Spradley (1979, 1980), Woods (1986) and others mention the building of typologies and taxonomies as an important component of analysis. Here the researcher aims to delineate subgroups within a general category. Such devices can become helpful in the identification of differences in the data and can help with the elucidation of relationships among concepts. Even the simplest of classifications, like Whyte's (1955) 'street corner' and 'college' boys, or Jenkins's (1983) 'lads', 'citizens' and 'ordinary kids', can help to organize amorphous material and to identify patterns in the data. Differences between the components of such classifications in terms of behaviour patterns are important in generating the kinds of linkages that will form the basis for the development of theory.

A particularly helpful discussion of analysis is provided by Bogdan and Biklen (1982), who distinguish between analysis in the field and analysis after data collection. Their approach owes much to grounded theory. In analysis in the field, the authors suggest that the researcher needs to be constantly engaging in preliminary analytic strategies during data collection. Such strategies include: forcing oneself to narrow down the focus of the study; continually reviewing field notes in order to determine whether new questions could fruitfully be asked; writing memos about what you have found out in relation to various issues (this is a grounded theory tactic); and trying out emergent ideas. Analysis after the field is essentially concerned with the development of a coding system. They present 'families of codes' which are fairly generic and can apply to a variety of different contexts. These include: setting/context codes; informants' perspectives; how informants think about people and objects; process codes; activity codes; strategy codes; and personal relationship codes.

A further classification of codes and coding has been provided by Miles and Huberman (1984), who distinguish between descriptive, interpretive, explanatory and astringent codes, these last being ones which 'pull a lot of material together' (p. 57). Lofland (1971) has provided a classification of 'social phenomena' which can usefully be employed as the basis for a coding scheme:

> Ranging from the microscopic to the macroscopic, these [social phenomena] are as follows:
> 1 *Acts.* Action in a situation that is temporally brief, consuming only a few seconds, minutes, or hours.
> 2 *Activities.* Action in a setting of more major duration – days, weeks, months – consuming significant elements of persons' involvements.
> 3 *Meanings.* The verbal production of participants that define and direct action.
> 4 Participation. Persons' holistic involvement in, or adaptation to, a situation or setting under study.
> 5 *Relationships.* Interrelationships among several persons considered simultaneously.
> 6 *Settings.* The entire setting under study conceived as the unit of analysis.   (1971: 14-15)

While there is a range of strategies and processes described in the texts, the question that arises is: How (if at all) are these used in practice? Some clues are provided in autobiographical writing, to which we now turn.

AUTOBIOGRAPHICAL ACCOUNTS

Among the most popular volumes devoted to research methodology in the last decade have been those which provide first person or autobiographical accounts where researchers have been invited to discuss the ways in which they actually conducted their research, in contrast to the ways they might be supposed to conduct it. Yet, even in these cases it is important to remember that it is post hoc reflections that are provided, with the result that projects are tidied up by their authors before being presented to a wider public. One of the first set of accounts to be provided in this genre was from the USA, where Hammond (1964) published *Sociologists at Work*. One of the great strengths of this volume was the way in which the various authors made links between theory and research. Indeed, in a subsequent evaluation of the essays in this volume, Baldamus (1972) highlights the importance of formal and informal theorizing, which has a bearing upon our theme of analysis. Within these early autobiographical essays authors describe the way in which they search for 'integrating principles', 'theoretical amalgams' and 'conceptual frameworks'. But we might ask: How does this link with data analysis?

Regrettably, there are few clues in the accounts which have been produced. In an editorial preface to a special issue of the journal *Urban Life and Culture* (now the *Journal of Contemporary Ethnography*), Lofland (1974) commented on the failings of autobiographical accounts. He considered that they provided little technical detail on the procedures associated with data collection and analysis. Instead, he argued that many accounts were little more than reviews of 'my adventures and nausea among the natives' (Lofland 1974: 307). In order to develop the level of discussion Lofland invited some successful fieldworkers (Cavan 1974, Davis 1974, Roth 1974, Wiseman 1974) to discuss data collection and analysis in one of their studies. To assist them in constructing their accounts, which would focus on procedures of data collection and analysis rather than on the social relations of fieldwork, he invited the researchers to address a set of questions. These included:

1   In what manner did you keep field and/or interview notes? Typed? Carbons? Dittoed? What was the rate of data accumulation, or waves of accumulation?
2   What workplace isolation or other place and physical devices did you employ to facilitate work on getting down material and working at its analysis?
3   How did you file, code or otherwise encode or sort the raw materials you accumulated? Marginal codes? Filing? Other?
4   How did the leading ideas that organized your present analysis evolve? A sudden flash? Slowly? Other?
5   What kinds of models or images are you aware of employing to organize the material? What were their sources?
6   To what degree did you organize your analysis before writing it out in text, versus writing it and then seeing what you had? Did you write a little every day, around the clock in bursts, or some other way?
7   In general, what were the most important difficulties and facilitants experienced in evolving the analysis and writing it up?
8   How would you, or have you, modified your practices since doing the particular work described here?   (Lofland 1974: 308)

While these questions focus on technical aspects of investigation, they should not be divorced from the social relations of fieldwork. The conduct of fieldwork is such that the social processes in which the fieldworker is engaged can have a direct influence on the modification of technical procedures and it is important for us to understand the dynamics of this relationship together with its implications for fieldwork.

Meanwhile, in Britain, Bell and Newby encouraged authors to contribute to the development of descriptive methodology through a series of accounts published under the title *Doing Sociological Research* (Bell and Newby 1977), in which authors were encouraged to write themselves into their accounts and to address such questions as:

> Why did you do this or that piece of research, when you did it in the way you did? How did you actually go about your research – what were the false starts, brilliant ideas and so on? What were the reactions, if any, to publication? What have been the personal consequences for you of the research?   (1977: 12)

Although the editors indicated that their list of questions was not exhaustive, it is evident that no explicit mention is made of analysis apart from a general reference to the way in which individuals went about research.

Authors such as Bell and Newby, and Bell and Encel (1978), moved us away from textbook procedures, and in doing so they tended to focus more upon research narrative rather than any of the technical aspects of social investigation. Indeed, it was the 1980s that witnessed increasing systematization from the authors of these accounts. However, the contributors to Roberts (1981) tended to focus more upon the way in which feminist research involved particular aspects of data collection that called for serious amendment. Interview approaches came under detailed scrutiny (Oakley 1981). Some of these themes were subsequently taken up in a volume edited by Bell and Roberts (1984), which pursued similar issues to those that both editors had been associated with in the recent past. Their earliest volumes were predominantly associated with data collection: participant observation and interviewing alongside several others.

Yet the editors of subsequent collections demonstrated some unease with this approach. For example, Burgess (1984b) devised a set of questions that his contributors might address in writing about their research practice. His questions demonstrate that issues concerning data analysis cannot be relegated to one simple section on the implications of various procedures for data analysis. Instead questions concerning analysis were raised throughout the research process. For example, when addressing matters of research access authors were invited to consider: 'How did these relationships [between sponsors and gatekeepers] influence data collection and analysis?' (p. 8). Similarly, analysis also figured in questions of language when he asked, 'What language skills were required in data collection and data analysis?'

(pp. 8-9). Such questions prefaced enquiries about data analysis which were summarized as follows:

> What was the relationship between data collection and data analysis? What were the informal processes involved in data analysis? What technical procedures were used for analyzing field data? What form did the writing up take?
>
> (Burgess 1984b: 9)

In addition, he invited authors to make links between theory and analysis when he asked, 'What was the relationship between theory, data collection and data analysis?' (p. 9).

Such questions point to the overlap between different aspects of the research process, with research access, data collection and data recording having implications for analysis, while analysis also links to the process of theorizing and writing. In the accounts that followed, authors demonstrated how analysis was not an activity to be relegated to the end of a research project, but was rather a central part of the continuous process of doing research. Several investigators demonstrated how the notes that were taken during a project were an important element in understanding the social structures under study (King 1984). The process of note taking was therefore highlighted not only as a means of data collection, but also as an important location for formal and informal analysis through commentary and coding.

Some authors demonstrated very clearly how analysis relates to formal and informal procedures, where themes emerge from data and from interview transcriptions (Porter 1984, Stenhouse 1984). Other strategies that are discussed involve looking for incidents (Delamont 1984) and the generation of theory from data using the model devised by Glaser and Strauss (1967). Yet sociologists have also been involved in devising new concepts in the course of conducting research so that data analysis gives rise to exploration and theory development.

Some of these procedures have been elaborated upon in other volumes (Burgess 1990, 1992), but many autobiographical essays remain silent on analysis in an explicit way. For example, Bryman (1988) encouraged his contributors to write about the formal and informal aspects of doing research in organizations, but he did not include analysis in his guide to topics on which his authors might write. Yet his volume contains an important essay by Turner (1988), who demonstrates the ways in which some of the principles associated with the work of Glaser and Strauss can be developed in practice.

Among the latest accounts in this genre is a collection of autobiographical accounts edited by Walford (1991), whose contributors focus on studies in education. While the volume continues to add to our knowledge of research practice, the focus is upon the practical and social aspects of conducting research. Accordingly, the editor tells us, 'all the chapters aim to share some of the challenges and embarrassments, the pains and triumphs, the ambiguities and satisfactions of trying to discover what is unknown' (1991: 5). As a consequence, there is a tendency to return to the story-telling mode of such essays, where a segment of the research process is scrutinized. Nevertheless, three qualitative essays do feature aspects of data analysis in an implicit or explicit way. For example, Measor and Woods (1991) tell us a little about analysis, since the main sections of their essay are devoted to research planning and design, access, and collaborative research. However, it is only in the subsection on writing that we get a glimpse of analysis through comments that Measor makes on an early draft of material written by Woods, where she talks of examples that are 'proof' of their analysis. Meanwhile, essays by Mercer (1991) and Ball (1991) give insights into the explicit processes associated with analysis in educational studies. In both instances they demonstrate that analysis is not a mere segment of the research process but is integral to other aspects of the conduct of investigation.

THE ORGANIZATION OF THIS VOLUME

The contributors to this volume were all invited to provide an exposition of the way in which they went about the analysis of qualitative data by providing a chapter in which there would be a balance between technical procedures and research examples. Our strategy was to issue invitations to those who had been involved in different kinds of qualitative investigations: studies based on the classic lone researcher approach, joint investigations, and research teams involved in multi-site studies, as well as studies that highlight the use of computers, policy issues and theorizing. Each of the contributors to this collection focuses on qualitative data analysis, but does so in his or her own way. Indeed, two essays that follow illustrate that there is no standard approach to the analysis of qualitative data; secondly, that data analysis relates not only to technical procedures but also to the social relations aspects of fieldwork; finally, that much of the work in which investigators engage in this phase of the research process is as much implicit as explicit.

Our collection opens with an essay from Judith Okely, an anthropologist who works within the classic tradition of ethnographic inquiry, but unlike the classical anthropologists such as Malinowski she focuses on the study of an aspect of her own society. Yet in this instance, the situation she was studying was simultaneously familiar (her own society) yet strange (the world of Gypsies) – an aspect of her work which had an important influence on her understanding and subsequent writing. The approach that was used by anthropologists has subsequently been taken up and developed by sociologists who have conducted ethnographic studies in schools, hospitals, factories and other social institutions. Yet it is relatively rare for the sociologist to move from public settings into the private domain of the family. But this is what Christina Hughes did in conducting a study of stepparents. Her chapter provides another example of the lone researcher developing insights from her fieldwork experience.

Alongside those studies conducted in anthropology and sociology that follow a classical approach, there is also a range of studies in a variety of social science disciplines utilizing more specialist approaches to qualitative data collection and analysis. Among the approaches used have been ethnomethodology, conversation analysis and discourse analysis. It is the last approach that is represented by Jonathan Potter and Margaret Wetherell so that comparisons can be made with the more conventional approaches. Indeed, a further major development in the social sciences has been the impact of feminism on data analysis. Accordingly, the chapter from Marilyn Poner discusses the role of team leader and illustrates the ways in which issues in feminist studies had an impact upon her analysis. Furthermore, although her chapter is single-authored, the study on which she is writing was produced by a team of social scientists.

It is this use of research teams that is explored through a series of chapters. First, by Jennifer Mason who was part of a two-member team. Here, she highlights the way in which she worked with her co-researcher to develop, collect, analyze and report data. In a further team-based chapter, Virginia Olesen and her co-investigators demonstrate much of the rich texture on the process of memo writing and exchange which assists in the development of analytic insights. Finally, a chapter from Robert Burgess and his team illustrates the way in which multi-site work can be developed through a systematic division of labour between team members, but where a discussion of key issues, insights and themes becomes essential for common conceptual development.

Certainly, conceptual development is a critical issue in the conduct of data analysis. In the final contributions to this volume, further themes are explored in this direction. First, the chapter from Lyn and Tom Richards discusses the development of conceptual themes on the basis of computer analysis. Second, there is a chapter from researchers in a qualitative research unit (Jane Ritchie and Liz Spencer) where interview-based studies are to the fore and topics and categories are extracted from transcripts for policy purposes as well as the development of social science. In a further contribution we turn to an essay by Barry Turner, who highlights the way in which thinking and theorizing are conducted in order to develop conceptual categories that will contribute to the social sciences as well as to our understanding of substantive fields. Finally, we provide some reflections on qualitative data analysis.

The essays that follow are therefore accounts of different approaches to data analysis in action. Together they illustrate that there is no standard approach but that a rich variety of approaches is characteristic of conducting qualitative research.

Notes

1   From the study by Jon Gubbay (University of East Anglia), personal communication.

Most frequently cited methods texts in undergraduate research methods courses in Britain 1990-1

Rank order	Citations
1 D. De Vaus, *Surveys in Social Research*	10
2 R.G. Burgess, *In the Field*	4
2 M. Hammersley and P. Atkinson, *Ethnography: Principles in Practice*	4
4 M. Bulmer (ed.), *Sociological Research Methods*	3
4 R.G. Burgess (ed.), *Field Research: a Sourcebook and Field Manual*	3
4 G. Rose, *Deciphering Sociological Research*	3
7 C. Bell and H. Roberts, *Social Researching*	2
7 A. Bryman, *Quantity and Quality in Social Research*	2
7 Frances Clegg, *Simple Statistics*	2
7 C. Marsh, The *Survey Method*	2
7 C. Marsh, *Exploring Data*	2
7 K. Plummer, *Documents of Life*	2
7 J. Scott, A *Matter of Record*	2
7 *Social Trends*	2

Notes:
(a)   These data are based on a study of 68 courses.
(b)   These texts were on lists which indicated students must read them in order to cope with the course.

2 It is not easy to specify how far coding in grounded theory and qualitative data analysis generally differs from that which takes place in quantitative data analysis. In part, this difficulty derives from an occasional tendency to caricature quantitative coding. Thus, Charmaz has written,

Qualitative coding is not the same as quantitative coding . . . . Quantitative coding requires preconceived, logically deduced codes into which the data are placed. Qualitative coding . . . means *creating* categories from interpretation of the data.
(1983: 111, emphasis in original)

However, this statement applies more to pre-coded questions in quantitative research or the coding of answers to open-ended questions to which an explicit coding frame can be applied in advance (which can be quite rare in social science research). Very often when conducting 'quantitative coding' of open-ended questions, a researcher has to create a coding frame out of an initial reading of the answers provided to the questions, so that at least the initial categorization has an emergent quality. The difference between this coding and that which occurs in grounded theory lies in the tendency for coding in qualitative data analysis to be more provisional (since conceptualization is under constant revision) and for codes to represent different levels of elaboration (some will be highly speculative; others, at a later stage of elaboration, will be more developed in terms of theoretical abstraction). In quantitative data analysis, codes become 'fixed' more rapidly and tend to be similar in terms of their level of theoretical development.

References

Atkinson, P. (1990) *The Ethnographic Imagination* London: Routledge.

Babbie, E.R. (1979) *The Practice of Social Research*, 2nd edn, Belmont, Calif.: Wadsworth.

Baldamus, W. (1972) 'The role of discoveries in social science', in T. Shanin (ed.) *The Rules of the Game*, London: Tavistock.

Ball, S.J. (1991) 'Power, conflict, micropolitics and all that!' in G. Walford (ed.) *Doing Educational Research*, London: Routledge.

Bechhofer, F. (1974) 'Current approaches to empirical research: some central ideas', in J. Rex (ed.) *Approaches to Sociology: an Introduction to Major Trends in British Sociology*, London: Routledge & Kegan Paul.

Bell, C. and Encel, S. (eds) (1978) *Inside the Whale*, Oxford: Pergamon.

Bell, C. and Newby, H. (eds) (1977) *Doing Sociological Research*, London: Allen & Unwin.

Bell, C. and Roberts, H. (eds) (1984) *Social Researching*, London: Routledge.

Bogdan, R.C. and Bikien, S.K. (1982) *Qualitative Research for Education*, Boston, Mass.: Allyn & Bacon.

Bogdan, R. and Taylor, S.J. (1975) *Introduction to Qualitative Research Methods*, New York: Wiley.

Bryman, A. (1988) *Quantity and Quality in Social Research*, London: Unwin Hyman.

Bulmer, M. (1979) 'Concepts in the analysis of qualitative data', *Sociological Review* 27: 651-77.

Bulmer, M. and Burgess, R.G. (eds) (1981) 'The teaching of research methodology', *Sociology* 15 (4) (special issue).

Burgess, R.G. (ed.) (1982) *Field Research: a Sourcebook and Field Manual*, London: Unwin Hyman.

- (1984a) *in the Field: an Introduction to Field Research*, London: Allen & Unwin.

- (ed.) (1984b) *The Research Process in Educational Settings: Ten Case Studies*, Lewes: Falmer Press.

- (ed.) (1989) *The Ethics of Educational Research*, Lewes, Falmer Press.

- (ed.) (1990) *Reflections on Field Experience*, London: JAI Press.

- (ed.) (1992) *Learning about Fieldwork*, London: JAI Press.

Cavan, 5. (1974) 'Seeing social structure in a rural setting', *Urban Life and Culture* 3(3): 329-46

Charmaz, K. (1983) 'The grounded theory method: an explication and interpretation' in R.M. Emerson (ed.) *Contemporary Field Research*, Boston, Mass.: Little, Brown.

Cicourel, A. (1964) *Method and Measurement in Sociology*, New York: Free Press.

Cressey, D. (1950) 'The criminal violation of personal trust', *American Sociological Review* 15: 738-43.

Davis, F. (1974) 'Stories and sociology', *Urban Life and Culture* 3(3): 310-16.

Delamont, 5. (1984) 'The old girl network: recollections on the fieldwork at St Luke's', in R.G. Burgess (ed.) *The Research Process in Educational Settings: Ten Case Studies*, Lewes: Falmer Press.

De Vaus, D. (1991) *Surveys in Social Research*, 2nd edn, London: UCL Press.

Fielding, N.G. and Lee, R.M. (eds) (1991) *Using Computers in Qualitative Research*, London: Sage.

Finch, J. (1986) *Research and Policy*, Lewes: Falmer Press.

Frankfort-Nachmias, C. and Nachmias, D. (1982) *Research Methods in the Social Sciences*, London: Edward Arnold.

Glaser, B.G. (1978) *Theoretical Sensitivity*, Mill Valley, Calif.: Sociology Press.

Glaser, B.G. and Strauss, A.L. (1967) *The Discovery of Grounded Theory: Strategies for Qualitative Research*, Chicago: Aldine.

Goetz, J.P. and Le Compte, M.D. (1984) *Ethnography and Qualitative Design in Educational Research*, Orlando, Fla.: Academic Press.

Hammersley , M. (1989) *The Dilemma of Qualitative Method: Herbert Blumer and the Chicago Tradition*, London: Routledge.

- (1991) *Reading Ethnography*, London: Longman.

-- (1992) *What's Wrong with Ethnography?*, London: Routledge.

Hammersley, M. and Atkinson, P. (1983) *Ethnography: Principles in Practice*, London: Tavistock.

Hammond, P. (ed.) (1964) *Sociologists at Work*, New York: Basic Books.

Jenkins, R. (1983) *Lads, Citizens, and Ordinary Kids: Working-Class Youth Styles in Belfast*, London: Routledge & Kegan Paul.

Kidder, L.H. and Judd, C.M. (1986) *Research Methods in Social Relations*, 5th edn, New York: Holt, Rinehart & Winston.

King, R. (1984) 'The man in the wendy house: researching infants schools', in R.G. Burgess (ed.) *The Research Process in Educational Settings: Ten Case Studies*, Lewes: Falmer Press.

Lindesmith, A.R. (1 947) *Opiate Addiction*, Bloomington, Ind.: Principle Press (published in 1968 as *Addiction and Opiates*, Chicago: Aldine).

Lofland, J. (1971) *Analyzing Social Settings: a Guide to Qualitative Observation and Analysis*, Belmont, Calif.: Wadsworth.

- (1974) 'Analyzing qualitative data: first person accounts', *Urban Life and Culture* 3(3): 307-9.

Marsh, C. (1979) 'Social sciences methods bibliography: British universities 1978', Cambridge: Social and Political Sciences Committee, University of Cambridge (mimeo).

Martin, P.Y. and Turner, B.A. (1986) 'Grounded theory and organizational research', *Journal of Applied Behavioural Science* 22: 141-58.

Measor, L. and Woods, P. (1991) 'Breakthroughs and blockages in ethnographic research: contrasting experiences during the changing schools project', in G. Walford (ed.) *Doing Educational Research*, London: Routledge.

Mercer, N. (1991) 'Researching common knowledge: studying the content and context of educational discourse', in G. Walford (ed.) *Doing Educational Research*, London: Routledge.

Miles, M.B. and Huberman, M. (1984) *Qualitative Data Analysis*, Beverley Hills, Calif.: Sage.

Moser, C.A. and Kalton, G. (1971) *Survey Methods in Social Investigation*, London: Heinemann.

Oakley, A. (1981) 'Interviewing women: a contradiction in terms', in H. Roberts (ed.) *Doing Feminist Research*, London: Routledge.

Oppenheim, A.N. (1966) *Questionnaire Design and Attitude Measurement*, London: Heinemann.

Peel, J. (1968) *Courses Mainly Concerned with Sociological Theory and Methods in 29 Universities*, 15th Conference of Sociology Teachers Section of the BSA, London: British Sociological Association.

Porter, M.A. (1984) 'The modification of method in researching postgraduate education', in R.G. Burgess (ed.) *The Research Process in Educational Settings: Ten Case Studies*, Lewes: Falmer Press.

Richards, L. and Richards, T. (1991) 'The transformation of qualitative method: computational paradigms and research processes', in N.G. Fielding and R.M. Lee (eds) *Using Computers in Qualitative Research*, London: Sage.

Roberts, H. (ed.) (1981) *Doing Feminist Research*, London: Routledge.

Robinson, W.S. (1951) 'The logical structure of analytic induction', *American Sociological Review* 16: 812-18.

Roth, J. (1974) 'Turning adversity to account', *Urban Life and Culture* 3(3): 347-59.

Seidel, J.V. and Clark, J.A. (1984) 'The Ethnograph: a computer program for the analysis of qualitative data', *Qualitative Sociology* 7:110-25.

Spradley, J.P. (1979) *The Ethnographic Interview*, New York: Hoit, Rinehart & Winston.

- (1980) *Participant Observation*, New York: Holt, Rinehart & Winston.

Stenhouse, L. (1984) 'Library use and user education in academic sixth fonms: an autobiographical account', in R.G. Burgess (ed.) *The Research Process in Educational Settings: Ten Case Studies*, Lewes: Falmer Press.

Strauss, A.L. (1987) *Qualitative Analysis for Social Scientists*, Cambridge and New York: Cambridge University Press.

Strauss, A.L. and Corbin, J. (1990) *Basics of Qualitative Research*, Newbury Park, Calif.: Sage.

Sutton, R.I. (1987) 'The process of organizational death: disbanding and reconnecting', *Administrative Science Quarterly* 32: 570-89.

Tesch, R. (1990) *Qualitative Research: Analytic Types and Software Tools*, Lewes: Falmer Press.

- (1991) 'Software for qualitative researchers: analysis needs and program capabilities', in N.G. Fielding and R.M. Lee (eds) *Using Computers in Qualitative Research*, London: Sage.

Turner, B.A. (1981) 'Some practical aspects of qualitative data analysis: one way of organising the cognitive processes associated with the generation of grounded theory', *Quality and Quantity* 15: 225-47.

- (1988) 'Connoisseurship in the study of organizational cultures', in A. Bryman (ed.) *Doing Research in Organizations*, London: Routledge.

Wakeford, J. (1979) 'Research Methods Syllabuses in Sociology Departments in the United Kingdom', Lancaster: Department of Sociology, University of Lancaster (mimeo).

Walford, G. (ed.) (1991) *Doing Educational Research*, London: Routledge.

Whyte, W.F. (1955) *Street Corner Society*, 2nd edn, Chicago: University of Chicago Press.

- *(1984) Lessons from the Field: a Guide from Experience*, Beverley Hills, Calif.: Sage.

Williams, R. (1976) 'Symbolic interactionism: fusion of theory and rrsearch', in D.C. Thorns (ed.) *New Directions in Sociology*, London: David & Charles.

Wiseman, J. (1974) 'The research web', *Urban Life and Culture 3 (3):* 317-28.

Woods, P. (1986) *Inside Schools: Ethnography in Educational Research*, London: Routledge.

This article was first published in the BMJ and is reproduced by permission of the BMJ.

This is the second of seven articles describing non-quantitative techniques and showing their value in health research

RIGOUR AND QUALITATIVE RESEARCH
Nicholas Mays, Catherine Pope

Nicholas Mays, *director of health services research* King's Fund Institute, London W2 4HT

Catherine Pope, *lecturer in social and behavioural medicine* Department of Epidemiology and Public Health, University of Leicester, Leicester LE1 6TP

BMJ 1995;311:109-12

Various strategies are available within qualitative research to protect against bias and enhance the reliability of findings. This paper gives examples of the principal approaches and summarises them into a methodological checklist to help readers of reports of qualitative projects to assess the quality of the research.

CRITICISMS OF QUALITATIVE RESEARCH

In the health field—with its strong tradition of biomedical research using conventional, quantitative, and often experimental methods—qualitative research is often criticised for lacking scientific rigour. To label an approach "unscientific" is peculiarly damning in an era when scientific knowledge is generally regarded as the highest form of knowing. The most commonly heard criticisms are, firstly, that qualitative research is merely an assembly of anecdote and personal impressions, strongly subject to researcher bias; secondly, it is argued that qualitative research lacks reproducibility—the research is so personal to the researcher that there is no guarantee that a different researcher would not come to radically different conclusions; and, finally, qualitative research is criticised for lacking generalisability. It is said that qualitative methods tend to generate large amounts of detailed information about a small number of settings.

IS QUALITATIVE RESEARCH DIFFERENT?

The pervasive assumption underlying all these criticisms is that quantitative and qualitative approaches are fundamentally different in their ability to ensure the validity and reliability of their findings. This distinction, however, is more one of degree than of type. The problem of the relation of a piece of research to some presumed underlying "truth" applies to the conduct of any form of social research. "One of the greatest methodological fallacies of the last half century in social research is the belief that science is a particular set of techniques; it is, rather, a state of mind, or attitude, and the organisational conditions which allow that attitude to be expressed."[1] In quantitative data analysis it is possible to generate statistical representations of phenomena which may or may not be fully justified since, just as in qualitative work, they will depend on the

judgment and skill of the researcher and the appropriateness to the question answered of the data collected. All research is selective—there is no way that the researcher can in any sense capture the literal truth of events. All research depends on collecting particular sorts of evidence through the prism of particular methods, each of which has its strengths and weaknesses. For example, in a sample survey it is difficult for the researcher to ensure that the questions, categories, and language used in the questionnaire are shared uniformly by respondents and that the replies returned have the same meanings for all respondents. Similarly, research that relies exclusively on observation by a single researcher is limited by definition to the perceptions and introspection of the investigator and by the possibility that the presence of the observer may, in some way that is hard to characterise, have influenced the behaviour and speech that was witnessed. Britten and Fisher summarise the position neatly by pointing out that "there is some truth in the quip that quantitative methods are reliable but not valid and that qualitative methods are valid but not reliable."[2]

STRATEGIES TO ENSURE RIGOUR IN QUALITATIVE RESEARCH

As in quantitative research, the basic strategy to ensure rigour in qualitative research is systematic and self conscious research design, data collection, interpretation, and communication. Beyond this, there are two goals that qualitative researchers should seek to achieve: to create an account of method and data which can stand independently so that another trained researcher could analyse the same data in the same way and come to essentially the same conclusions; and to produce a plausible and coherent explanation of the phenomenon under scrutiny. Unfortunately, many qualitative researchers have neglected to give adequate descriptions in their research reports of their assumptions and methods, particularly with regard to data analysis. This has contributed to some of the criticisms of bias from quantitative researchers.

Yet the integrity of qualitative projects can be protected throughout the research process. The remainder of this paper discusses how qualitative researchers attend to issues of validity, reliability, and generalisability.

Sampling

Much social science is concerned with classifying different "types" of behaviour and distinguishing the "typical" from the "atypical." In quantitative research this concern with similarity and difference leads to the use of statistical sampling so as to maximise external validity or generalisability. Although statistical sampling methods such as random sampling are relatively uncommon in qualitative investigations, there is no reason in principle why they cannot be used to provide the raw material for a comparative analysis, particularly when the researcher has no compelling a prior reason for a purposive approach. For example, a random sample of practices could be studied in an investigation of how and why teamwork in primary health care is more and less successful in different practices. However, since qualitative data collection is generally more time consuming and expensive than, for example, a quantitative survey, it is not usually practicable to use a probability sample. Furthermore, statistical representativeness is not a prime requirement when the objective is to understand social processes.

An alternative approach, often found in qualitative research and often misunderstood in medical circles, is to use systematic, non-probabilistic sampling. The purpose is not to establish a random or representative sample drawn from a population but rather to identify specific groups of people who either possess characteristics or live in circumstances relevant to the social phenomenon being studied. Informants are identified because they will enable exploration of a particular aspect of behaviour relevant to the research. This approach to sampling allows the researcher deliberately to include a wide range of types of informants and also to select key informants with access to important sources of knowledge.

"Theoretical" sampling is a specific type of non-probability sampling in which the objective of developing theory or explanation guides the process of sampling and data collection.[3] Thus, the analyst makes an initial selection of informants; collects, codes, and analyses the data; and produces a preliminary theoretical explanation before deciding which further data to collect and from whom. Once these data are analysed, refinements are made to the theory, which may in turn guide further sampling and data collection. The relation between sampling and explanation is iterative and theoretically led.

To return to the example of the study of primary care team working, some of the theoretically relevant characteristics of general practices affecting variations in team working might be the range of professions represented in the team, the frequency of opportunities for communication among team members, the local organisation of services, and whether the practice is in an urban, city, or rural area. These factors could be identified from other similar research and within existing social science theories of effective and ineffective team working and would then be used explicitly as sampling categories. Though not statistically representative of general practices, such a sample is theoretically informed and relevant to the research questions. It also minimises the possible bias arising from selecting a sample on the basis of convenience.

Ensuring the reliability of an analysis

In many forms of qualitative research the raw data are collected in a relatively unstructured form such as tape recordings or transcripts of conversations. The main ways in which qualitative researchers ensure the retest reliability of their analyses is in maintaining meticulous records of interviews and observations and by documenting the process of analysis in detail. While it is possible to analyse such data singlehandedly and use ways of classifying and categorising the data which emerge from the analysis and remain implicit, more explicit group approaches, which perhaps have more in common with the quantitative social sciences, are increasingly used. The interpretative procedures are often decided on before the analysis. Thus, for example, computer software is available to facilitate the analysis of the content of interview transcripts.[4] A coding frame can be developed to characterise each utterance (for example, in relation to the age, sex, and role of the speaker; the topic; and so on), and transcripts can then be coded by more than one researcher.[5] One of the advantages of audiotaping or videotaping is the opportunity the tapes offer for subsequent analysis by independent observers.

The reliability of the analysis of qualitative data can be enhanced by organising an independent assessment of transcripts by additional skilled qualitative researchers and comparing agreement between the raters. For example, in a study of clinical encounters between cardiologists and their patients which looked at the differential value each derived from the information provided by echocardiography, transcripts of the clinic interviews were analysed for content and structure by the principal researcher and by an independent panel, and the level of agreement was assessed.[6]

Safeguarding validity

Alongside issues of reliability, qualitative researchers give attention to the validity of their findings. "Triangulation" refers to an approach to data collection in which evidence is deliberately sought from a wide range of different, independent sources and often by different means (for instance, comparing oral testimony with written records). This approach was used to good effect in a qualitative study of the effects of the introduction of general management into the NHS. The accounts of doctors, managers, and patient advocates were explored in order to identify patterns of convergence between data sources to see whether power relations had shifted appreciably in favour of professional managers and against the medical profession.[7]

Validation strategies sometimes used in qualitative research are to feed the findings back to the participants to see if they regard the findings as a reasonable account of their experience[8] and to use interviews or focus groups with

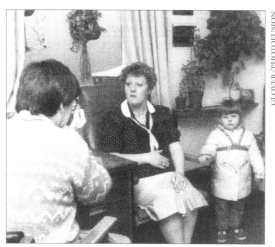

The differences in GPs' interviews with patients of handicapped and non-handicapped children have been shown by qualitative methods.

the same people so that their reactions to the evolving analysis become part of the emerging research data.[9] If used in isolation these techniques assume that fidelity to the participants' commonsense perceptions is the touchstone of validity. In practice, this sort of validation has to be set alongside other evidence of the plausibility of the research account since different groups are likely to have different perspectives on what is happening.[10]

A related analytical and presentational issue is concerned with the thoroughness with which the researcher examines "negative or "deviant" cases—those in which the researcher's explanatory scheme appears weak or is contradicted by the evidence. The researcher should give a fair account of these occasions and try to explain why the data vary.[11] In the same way, if the findings of a single case study diverge from those predicted by a previously stated theory, they can be useful in revising the existing theory in order to increase its reliability and validity.

Validity and explanation

It is apparent in qualitative research, particularly in observational studies (see the next paper in this series for more on observational methods), that the researcher can be regarded as a research instrument.[12] Allowing for the inescapable fact that purely objective observation is not possible in social science, how can the reader judge the credibility of the observer's account? One solution is to ask a set of questions: how well does this analysis explain why people behave in the way they do; how comprehensible would this explanation be to a thoughtful participant in the setting; and how well does the explanation it advances cohere with what we already know?

This is a challenging enough test, but the ideal test of a qualitative analysis, particularly one based on observation, is that the account it generates should allow another person to learn the "rules" and language sufficiently well to be able to function in the research setting. In other words, the report should carry sufficient conviction to enable someone else to have the

same experience as the original observer and appreciate the truth of the account.[13] Few readers have the time or inclination to go to such lengths, but this provides an ideal against which the quality of a piece of qualitative work can be judged.

The development of "grounded theory"[3] offers another response to this problem of objectivity. Under the strictures of grounded theory, the findings must be rendered through a systematic account of a setting that would be clearly recognisable to the people in the setting (by, for example, recording their words, ideas, and actions) while at the same time being more structured and self consciously explanatory than anything that the participants themselves would produce.

Attending to the context

Some pieces of qualitative research consist of a case study carried out in considerable detail in order to produce a naturalistic account of everyday life. For example, a researcher wishing to observe care in an acute hospital around the clock may not be able to study more than one hospital. Again the issue of generalisability, or what can be learnt from a single case, arises. Here, it is essential to take care to describe the context and particulars of the case study and to flag up for the reader the similarities and differences between the case study and other settings of the same type. A related way of making the best use of case studies is to show how the case study contributes to and fits with a body of social theory and other empirical work.[12] The final paper in this series discusses qualitative case studies in more detail.

Collecting data directly

Another defence against the charge that qualitative research is merely impressionistic is that of separating the evidence from secondhand sources and hearsay from the evidence derived from direct observation of behaviour in situ. It is important to ensure that the observer has had adequate time to become thoroughly familiar with the milieu under scrutiny and that the participants have had the time to become accustomed to having the researcher around. It is also worth asking whether the observer has witnessed a wide enough range of activities in the study site to be able to draw conclusions about typical and atypical forms of behaviour—for example, were observations undertaken at different times? The extent to which the observer has succeeded in establishing an intimate understanding of the research setting is often shown in the way in which the subsequent account shows sensitivity to the specifics of language and its meanings in the setting.

Minimising researcher bias in the presentation of results

Although it is not normally appropriate to write up qualitative research in the conventional format of the scientific paper, with a rigid distinction between the results and discussion sections of the account, it is important that the presentation of the research allows the reader as far as possible to distinguish the data, the analytic framework used, and the interpretation.[1] In quantitative research these distinctions are conventionally and neatly presented in the methods section, numerical tables, and the accompanying commentary. Qualitative research depends in much larger part on producing a convincing account.[14] In trying to do this it is all too easy to construct a narrative that relies on the reader's trust in the integrity and fairness of the researcher. The equivalent in quantitative research is to present tables of data setting out the statistical relations between operational definitions of variables without giving any idea of how the phenomena they represent present themselves in naturally occurring settings.[1] The need to quantify can lead to imposing arbitrary categories on complex phenomena, just as data extraction in qualitative research can be used selectively to tell a story that is rhetorically convincing but scientifically incomplete.

The problem with presenting qualitative analyses objectively is the sheer volume of data customarily available and the relatively greater difficulty faced by the researcher in summarising qualitative data. It has been suggested that a full transcript of the raw data should be made available to the reader on microfilm or computer disk,[11] although this would be cumbersome. Another partial solution is to present extensive sequences from the original data (say, of conversations), followed by a detailed commentary.

Another option is to combine a qualitative analysis with some quantitative summary of the results. The quantification is used merely to condense the results to make them easily intelligible; the approach to the analysis remains qualitative since naturally occurring events identified on theoretical grounds are being counted. The table shows how Silverman compared the format of the doctor's initial questions to parents in a paediatric cardiology clinic when the child was not handicapped with a smaller number of cases when the child had Down's syndrome. A minimum of interpretation was needed to contrast the two sorts of interview.[15 16]

Assessing a piece of qualitative research

This short paper has shown some of the ways in which researchers working in the qualitative tradition have endeavoured to ensure the rigour of their work. It is hoped that this summary will help the prospective reader of reports of qualitative research to identify some of the key questions to ask when trying to assess its quality. A range of helpful checklists has been published to assist readers of quantitative research assess the design[17] and statistical[18] and economic[19] aspects of individual published papers and review articles.[20] Likewise, the contents of this paper have been condensed into a checklist for readers of qualitative studies, covering design, data collection, analysis, and reporting (box). We hope that the checklist will give readers of studies in health and health care research that use qualitative methods the confidence to subject them to critical scrutiny.

Questions to ask of a qualitative study

- Overall, did the researcher make explicit in the account the theoretical framework and methods used at every stage of the research?
- Was the context clearly described?
- Was the sampling strategy clearly described and justified?
- Was the sampling strategy theoretically comprehensive to ensure the generalisability of the conceptual analyses (diverse range of individuals and settings, for example)?
- How was the fieldwork undertaken? Was it described in detail?
- Could the evidence (fieldwork notes, interview transcripts, recordings, documentary analysis, etc) be inspected independently by others; if relevant, could the process of transcription be independently inspected?
- Were the procedures for data analysis clearly described and theoretically justified? Did they relate to the original research questions? How were themes and concepts identified from the data?
- Was the analysis repeated by more than one researcher to ensure reliability?
- Did the investigator make use of quantitative evidence to test qualitative conclusions where appropriate?
- Did the investigator give evidence of seeking out observations that might have contradicted or modified the analysis?
- Was sufficient of the original evidence presented systematically in the written account to satisfy the sceptical reader of the relation between the interpretation and the evidence (for example, were quotations numbered and sources given)?

Form of doctor's questions to parents at a paediatric cardiology clinic[15]

Question	No of times asked
Random sample of children without handicap (n=22):	
Is he/she well?	11
From your point of view, is he/she a well baby?	2
Do you notice anything wrong with her/him?	1
From the heart point of view, she/he's active?	1
How is he/she?	4
Question not asked	3
Children with Down's syndrome (n = 12):	
Is he/she well?	0
From your point of view, is he/she a well baby?	1
Do you notice anything wrong with her/him?	0
As far as his/her heart is concerned, does he/she get breathless?	1
Does she/he get a few chest infections?	1
How is he/she (this little boy/girl) in himself/herself?	6
Question not asked	3

Further reading

Hammersley M. *Reading ethnographic research*. London: Longman, 1990.

References

1 Dingwall R. 'Don't mind him – he's from Barcelona': qualitative methods in health studies. In: Daly J, MacDonald I, Willis E, eds. *Researching health care: designs, dilemmas, disciplines.* London: Tavistock/Routledge, 1992: 161-75.

2 Britten N, Fisher B. Qualitative research and general practice [editorial]. *BrJ Gen Pract* 1993;**43**:270-1.

3 Glaser BG, Strauss AL. *The discovery of grounded theory.* Chicago: Aldine, 1967.

4 Seidel J, Clark JA. The ethnograph: a computer program for the analysis of qualitative data. *Qualitative Sociology* 1984;**7**:110-25.

5 Krippendorff K. Content analysis: an introduction to its metholology. London: Sage: 1980.

6 Daly J, MacDonald I, Willis E. Why don't you ask them? A qualitative research framework for investigating the diagnosis of cardiac normality. In: Daly J, MacDonald I, Willis E, eds. *Researching health care: designs, dilemmas, disciplines.* London: Tavistock/Routledge, 1992:189-206.

7 Pollitt C, Harrison S, Hunter DJ, Marnoch G. No hiding place: on the discomforts of researching the contemporary policy process. *Journal of Social Policys* 1990;**19**:169-90.

8 McKeganey NP, Bloor MJ. On the retrieval of sociological descriptions: respondent validation and the critical case of ettinomethodology. *International Journal of Sociology and Social Policy* 1981;**1**:58-69.

9 Oakley A. *The sociology of housework.* Oxford: Martin Robertson, 1974.

10 Brannen J. Combining qualitative and quantitative approaches: an overview. In: *Mixing methods: qualitative and quantitative research.* Aldershot: Avebury, 1992:3-37.

11 Waitzkin H. On studying the discourse of medical encounters: a critique of quantitative and qualitative methods and a proposal for reasonable compromise. *Med Care* 1990;**28**:473-88.

12 Mechanic D. Medical sociology: some tensions among theory, method and substance. *J Health Soc Behav* 1989;**30**:147-60.

13 Fielding N. Ethnography. In: Gilbert N, ed. *Researching social life.* London: Sage, 1993, 154-71.

14 Silverman D. Telling convincing stories: a plea for cautious positivism in case studies. In: Glassner B, Moreno J, eds. *The qualitative-quantitative distinction in the social sciences.* Dordrecht: Kluwer, 1989:57-77.

15 Silverman D. Applying the qualitative method to clinical care. In: Daly J, MacDonald I, Willis E, eds. *Researching health care: designs, dilemmas, disciplines.* London: Tavistock/Routledge, 1992:176-88.

16 Silverman D. The child as a social object: Down's syndrome children in a paediatric cardiology clinic. *Sociology of Health and Illness* 1981;**3**:254-74.

17 Fowkes FGR, Fulton PM. Critical appraisal of published research: introductory guidelines. *BMJ* 1991;**302**:1136-40.

18 Gardner MJ, Machin D, Campbell MJ. Use of check lists in assessing the statistical content of medical studies. *BMJ* 1986;**292**:810-2.

19 Department of Clinical Epidemiology and Biostatistics. How to read clinical journals. VII. To understand an economic evaluation (part B). *Can Med Assoc J* 1984;**130**:1542-9.

20 Oxman AD, Guyatt GH. Guidelines for reading literature reviews. *Can Med Assoc J* 1988;**138**:697-703.

This article was first published in Family Practice (Oxford University Press) and is reproduced by permission of Oxford University Press

A REVIEW OF RECENTLY PUBLISHED QUALITATIVE RESEARCH IN GENERAL PRACTICE. MORE METHODOLOGICAL QUESTIONS THAN ANSWERS?

Pat Hoddinott and Roisin Pill

Received 4 December 1996; Accepted 3 April 1997.

Department of General Practice, Health Centre, Llanedeyrn, Cardiff CF3 7PN, UK.

Pat Hoddinott is a general practitioner, and Roisin Pill is a social scientist and professor of research.

Family Practice 1997; **14**: 313–319.

Objective. This study aimed to review published papers which use qualitative interviewing in general practice as their methodology. To look specifically at the detail of how the methodology is presented to the reader, with particular emphasis on the clarity of detail about recruitment, the relationship of the interviewer to the respondents, the setting and how the research was presented to the respondents.

Methods and results. A systematic search using *Medline* and hand searching the *British Journal of General Practice, Family Practice* and *Social Science and Medicine* identified 29 recent papers using qualitative interviewing techniques in general practice. The papers were analysed for eight methodological criteria by the author. A second analysis, blind to the results of the first analysis was performed by the author 6 weeks later. An independent assessor analysed 12 randomly selected papers. There was 98.3% intra-assessor agreement and 89.6% inter-assessor agreement about whether the eight criteria were met. Overall 140 of a possible 232 criteria were met (60.3%).

Conclusion. Published papers using qualitative interviewing in general practice often lack explicit methodological detail about the relationship between the interviewer and the respondents, the setting, who did the recruiting and how the research was explained to the respondents. This methodological detail is important for the critical appraisal of qualitative research, where the context of the research can influence the data.

Keywords. General practice, interviewing, methodology, qualitative research.

INTRODUCTION

Qualitative methods are being increasingly promoted as appropriate for general practice research.[1-4] However, qualitative research in general practice is seldom published and guidelines for authors submitting papers for publication are orientated towards quantitative methodologies. In qualitative research the aim is to gain understanding of a topic from the respondents' perspective. The relationship between the subject and the interviewer, together with the context in which the interviews take place, are important details in appraising qualitative research. A published paper should provide sufficient methodological detail for a reader to be able to replicate the study and confirm the findings if required.

The author is currently undertaking a qualitative study in general practice, looking at the infant feeding decision making process for women expecting their first baby. This study arose from a debate about whether to interview women as a GP or as an unknown researcher and is discussed in a separate paper (this issue). To inform this debate, a systematic review of published papers using qualitative methods in general practice was performed to see how other researchers have addressed the methodological issues arising from the relationship between the interviewer and the respondents.

METHODS

Papers published between January 1992 and October 1996 which used qualitative interview methodology in general practice were identified by a *Medline* literature search. The textwords 'qualitative' 'general practice' 'interview' and 'primary care' were searched to identify relevant papers. This was complemented by hand searching in the *British Journal of General Practice, Family Practice* and *Social Science and Medicine*. These particular journals were identified as being most likely to publish qualitative research in general practice, and to identify the number of papers missed by *Medline*. Papers were only included if the respondents were recruited from a general practice population or the qualitative interviewer was a GP. Research studies using focus groups alone were not included. Papers were excluded where the respondents were health professionals or where ordinary consultations were used, with no additional data collection agenda. Papers which were predominantly quantitative in design and using structured interviews were also excluded. Each paper was systematically analysed for the following criteria: (i) were the qualifications and professional roles of the researchers clearly stated?; (ii) was it clear who did the interviewing?; (iii) how were the respondents recruited?; (iv) who recruited the respondents and what was their relationship to the respondents and to the interviewer?; (v) were the authors explicit about how the research topic was explained to the respondents?; (vi) was the interviewer known to the respondents and how did the interviewer introduce himself/herself?; (vii) where did the interviews

Table 1
Published papers using qualitative interviewing in general practice in four peer-reviewed journals and whether eight methodological criteria were met

Methodological criteria used for assessing papers	Br Med J (n = 6)[6-11]	Br J Gen Pract (n - 11)[12-22]	Fam Pract (n = 9)[5,23-30]	Soc Sci Med (n = 3)[31-33]
Researcher details given	6	10	2	1
Interviewer details given	5	9	5	2
Explicit about how recruited	6	11	9	3
Explicit about who did recruiting	4	6	4	1
Research topic explicit	4	5	2	2
Explicit about whether interviewer known and how introduced	2	4	2	1
Setting of interviews stated	4	10	8	2
Methodological issues raised	4	2	4	0

take place?; and (viii) were the methodological issues about the influence of the interviewer's role on the data discussed?

The papers were initially analysed on two separate occasions by the author. The analyses were performed approximately 6 weeks apart and the second analysis was performed without reference to the results of the first analysis. To check reliability of the analysis, a computer-generated random sample of 12 of the papers was independently and blindly analysed for the eight criteria by a senior lecturer in general practice.

RESULTS

Twenty-nine articles were identified, 18 by *Medline* and 11 by hand searching. Four of the papers identified by hand searching were too recent to be on *Medline*. Of the other papers identified by hand searching, five were from *Family Practice* and two were from the *British Journal of General Practice*.

Overall 140 of a possible 232 criteria were met (60.3%). Tables 1 and 2 show the number of papers that met the defined methodological criteria. There was 98.3% (228 of 232 items) agreement between the two analyses performed by the author and 89.6% agreement (86 of 96 items) between the author and the independent assessor. Disagreement occurred mainly about the clarity of the researchers' roles and qualifications. It was felt that they should be clear enough to be able to make an assessment about how the data might be influenced by the researchers and their particular perspective. Other areas of disagreement occurred when methodological information arose for the first time in the discussion part of the paper. Criteria where disagreement occurred are marked on Table 2.

In 11 papers a GP was definitely the interviewer. In five of these papers the respondents were the GP's own patients, in three papers it was unclear, and in three papers the GP interviewed respondents who were not patients. Only one paper discusses in detail the methodological issue of combining the role of qualitative interviewer with being a OP and the effect it had on the study.[5] Many ambiguities about the roles of the researchers arose due to the use of the third person

in reporting the research. This style is used to convey objectivity in reporting quantitative research, but is not always appropriate in reporting qualitative research, where depth of understanding is paramount and the relationship between the researcher and the respondent is an important part of the methodology. Kai uses the first person singular in reporting his methodology to avoid ambiguity and his two recent papers were the only ones to fulfil all eight methodological criteria.[6,7]

CONCLUSION

This review highlights an important lack of contextual detail in published papers which use qualitative research methods in general practice. Too often the reader has to make assumptions about the finer details of the design or have personal knowledge about the qualifications of the researcher. Each qualitative study is unique in design and analysis, and depends on the skills and perspectives of the researcher. Without rigorous reporting of methodology it becomes difficult to critically appraise qualitative research. It is not known to what extent omissions may be due to editorial decisions rather than the authors.

Qualitative research in general practice is still in its infancy. There are gaps in the methodological literature which are hotly debated, particularly whether GPs should interview their own patients. New researchers to the field are likely to turn to existing studies for information about design and relevant methodological issues: at the moment they are likely to be disappointed by the lack of explicit detail and discussion of this issue. Authors and editors of qualitative research papers for publication in medical journals need clear guidelines about the methodological detail required.

ACKNOWLEDGEMENTS

We would like to thank Dr Paul Kinnersley for acting as independent assessor of a sample of the papers and to Dr Paul Kinnersley and Dr Chris Butler for their helpful comments on the paper. Dr Pat Hoddinott has a Royal College of General Practitioners Research Training Fellowship which has helped fund her research.

Table 2

Published papers using qualitative interviewing in general practice and whether eight defined methodological criteria were met

Paper	Researchers' roles and qualifications clear?	Interviewer details given?	Explicit about how respondents were recruited?	Explicit about who recruited the respondents?	Explicit about how the research was explained to the respondents?	Explicit about whether interviewer known to respondents and how introduced?	Interview setting stated?	Were methodological issues about the influence of the interviewer on the data addressed?
Murphy, Kinmonth and Marteau[21]	Yes. Researcher, reader in general practice and psychologist	Yes. Researcher	Yes. From two general practices	Yes. Letter signed by their GP and consultant and telephoned by interviewer	No	No. Assume not known from reading paper	Yes. At home	No
Kai[9]	[a]Yes. Lecturer in primary care	Yes. GP	Yes. Opportunistic from baby clinic	No	No	No. Not explicit. Assume that they are known from reading paper	Yes. At home and the surgery	No
Borkan, Shvartzman, Reis and Morris[24]	No. GPs. Roles of other authors unknown	Yes. GPs	Yes. Convenience sample of patients presenting at clinic for medical care	No	Yes. Asked to provide stories of their experiences during war	No. Not explicit about whether GP known to patients	Yes. Clinics	No
Cornford, Morgan and Ridsdale[25]	No. ? GPs	No. Unclear. Pilot interviews done by one author	Yes. Consecutive recruitment by GP in neighbouring practice. Letter or telephone	Yes. A GP, but no details of who sent recruitment letter or telephoned patients	No	No. Explicit only about pilot interviews which were done in GP's own practice	Yes. At home	No
Brorrson and Rastam[26]	No. One a GP but role of other author unknown	Yes. GP	Yes. Strategic sampling from consultations	No	No	No	Yes. Primary care consultations	No
Murray and Shepherd[31]	No. One a research worker. Place of work stated	Yes. Interviewer a research worker	[a]Yes. Respondents selected from questionnaire in earlier part of study	No. Not clear – assume from reading paper that the authors did the recruiting	No	No	No	No

ARTICLE 15

Article 15

Study								
Fisher and Britten[20]	Yes. GP + social scientist	Yes. GP	Yes. Telephoned by interviewer	Yes	No. Assume from reading that it was explicit	[a]Yes. Mentioned in discussion but not in methods	Yes. At home	Yes. Mentions the difference in patient response. Does not mention GP in two roles
Britten[12]	Yes. Lecturer in medical sociology	Yes. Lecturer in medical sociology	Yes. Attenders and non-attenders at two GP practices	Yes. Introductory letter signed by GP or practice manager	Yes. Patients' ideas about medicines and treatment	No	Yes. At home except three	No
Hamberg, Johansson, Lindgren and Westman[5]	No. Two authors GPs (stated in text but not with title). Other two unclear. One from a department of sociology	Yes. GPs	Yes. Explicit in recruiting women who agreed to be interviewed and have interviewers as their GP	Yes. The GPs met with subjects prior to the study	No. Not explicitly stated. Assume that they were explicit from reading paper	Yes. Pros and cons discussed	No	Yes. Pros and cons discussed including the difficulty of having two roles
Jones and Greenwood[17]	Yes. GP and anthropologist	Yes. Interviews by an anthropologist	Yes	Yes. By GPs	Yes. Respondents asked to tell their story. Research agenda was to identify causes of distress	No. Assume from reading paper not known	Yes. At home	No
Kai[23]	Yes. GP (not mentioned until discussion)	Yes. GP. Not mentioned until the discussion section of the paper	Yes. Opportunistic from baby clinic	No	No	Yes. Not stated in methods but mentioned in discussion	Yes. At home and the surgery	Yes. Influence of interviewer being a known GP briefly mentioned
Britten[27]	No. Only place of work stated	No. The author	Yes. Attenders from appointment sheets. Non-attenders identified by practice manager	Yes. Letters signed by practice manager or GP	No	No	Yes. At home except three	No
Ridsdale and Hudd[18]	Yes. Senior lecturer and psychologist, department of general practice	Yes. Psychologist	Yes. Selected from appointment book and telephoned	No	No	Yes. Unknown to patients	Yes. At home	No

Mellor and Chambers[13]	Yes. GP and qualitative health researcher	Yes. External qualitative health researcher	No. At antenatal clinic, but no details of sampling methods	Yes. Recruited by midwives	Yes. Views on antenatal care and infant health care	Yes. Unknown to patients. Assume GP/ author's own practice	Yes. Practice interviews. Focus groups outside practice	No. Patients and practice working together to improve care discussed
Carman and Britten[14]	Yes. GP and social scientist	Yes. GP	Yes. Recruited by letter	No. No details of who signed recruiting letter	No	No. Went to practice where not known. Unclear how he was introduced. Discussion implies that he was introduced as a GP	a,bYes. At home	Yes. Mentions possible bias of respondents saying what they think the interviewer wants to hear
Dicker and Armstrong[8]	aYes. GP and social scientist	Yes. GP	No	No	Yes – handout with invitation	No. Not explicitly stated. Assume own patients from reading the paper	Yea. At the surgery	Yes. Discusses bias of GP interviewer
Lewis and Williamson[16]	aYes. Research worker and director of a health and social policy research centre	No. Interviews by a researcher	Yes. Consecutive patients after seeing a receptionist	No	Yes. Critical incident technique explained	bNo	Yes. In the practice	No
Murphy and Kinmonth[28]	No. Places of work stated, but not qualifications or roles	No	Yes. All diabetic patients on register of 8 GPs	Yes. GP letter introducing researcher	aYes. Asked to tell their story about their diabetes	No. Not explicitly stated whether interviewer known (assume not from text)	aYes. At home except one	No
Brorsson, Trocin, Lindbladh, Selander, Widlund and Rastam[29]	No. One author is a nurse and interviewer. Other authors – place of work stated but not qualifications	Yes. Nurse	Yes. Recruited from a health survey in a primary care centre	No	No. Presented as a counselling session on risks of high cholesterol. Not clear whether explicit about family history aim	bNo. Not clear whether nurse/ interviewer was known to the patients	Yes. Primary care centre	Yes. Interviewer a nurse rather than a doctor may have facilitated expression of ideas

ARTICLE 15

Study								
Whittaker[30]	Yes. Author part of a team of GPs and 3 anthropologists	No. Team approach unclear who did what	Yes. Snowball sampling of local community groups	No	[b]No. Unclear	No. Two participant observers living in the community. Not clear whether one was a GP or whether own patients	Yes. Majority at home	[a]Yes. Mention the different frameworks of GPs and anthropologists – similarities and differences
Borkan, Reis, Hermonia and Biderman[32]	No. Qualifications not mentioned, just place of work	No. Not explicitly stated	Yes. Purposeful sampling of patients known by OP and nurses in practice areas of the researchers	No. Identified by physicians and nurses, but not clear if recruited by them	Yes. Asked to present their story about their back pain	No	Yes. General practice surgery	No. Discusses the possible sample bias towards articulate respondents
Punamaki and Kokko[33]	Yes. 1 author an outside researcher, 1 author GP	Yes. Outside researcher	Yes. Patients at a week-end surgery - recruited by receptionist	Yes. Receptionist	Yes. To improve understanding of health and illness	Yes. Unknown researcher and unknown GP	Yes. General practice surgery	No. Mentions clinical setting as a drawback
Cunningham-Burley, Allbutt, Garraway, Lee and Russell[19]	No. Place of work and qualifications given. Unclear if any are GPs	[a]No. One of the authors with BA, MSc qualifications	Yes. Sample of patients from a GP surgery by letter	No. No details of who letter from	No	No	Yes. At home or convenient location	No
Skelton, Murphy and O'Dowd[15]	Yes. Two authors from a school of education, one social scientist and one GP	Yes. Interviewer from a school of education	Yes. Recruited by GPs from consultations	Yes. GPs	No	No. Assume not known from reading paper	No	No
Benson and Britten[11]	Yes. GP and lecturer in medical sociology	Yes. GP	Yes. Computer records of cancer patients	Yes. Authors, but no details of how invited and whether known to patients	No	No. Not explicit about whether GPs own practice or not	No	No
Cromarty[22]	Yes. RAF senior medical officer	Yes. A doctor presented as an interviewer, presumably the author	Yes. A random sample of video consultations from 11 GPs	No	Yes. Not known to respondents. Introduced as an interviewer	Yes. Respondents asked for their recollections	Yes. At home	No

Kai[7]	Yes. Lecturer in primary care	Yes. GP	Yes. Recruited from a range of community settings. Purposeful sampling	Yes. Invited to participate by a community worker	Yes. Discuss what was important to them when coping with ill young children	Yes. Knew he was a doctor - not his own patients. Pilot interviews - own patients	Yes. At home	Yes. There may have been bias towards discussing medical concepts rather than lay concepts
Kai[6]	Yes. Lecturer in primary care	Yes. GP	Yes. Recruited from a range of community settings. Purposeful sampling	Yes. Invited to participate by a community worker	Yes. Discuss what was important to them when coping with ill young children	Yes. Knew he was a doctor – not his own patients. Pilot interviews – own patients	Yes. At home	Yes. There may have been bias towards discussing medical concepts rather than lay concepts
Hopton, Hogg and McKee[10]	Yes. Research psychologist, health visitor and GP	No. State that 'we interviewed' implying the authors: all or some?	Yes. Random sample of out-of-hours calls from one practice	Yes. The authors sent a letter, but not explicit whether the authors worked in the practice	Yes. How people make decisions about health care. Unclear if the out-of-hours call was mentioned	No. Not explicit about whether interviewers worked in the practice from which respondents were being recruited	No	Yes. Respondents may have interpreted the interview as a request to justify the out-of-hours call

[a] Disagreement between independent assessor and author.

[b] Disagreement between two independent assessments by author.

References

[1] Britten N, Fisher B. Qualitative research and general practice. *Br J Gen Pract* 1993; **43**: 270–271.

[2] Shanks J, Kheray S, Fish S. Better ways of assessing health needs in primary care. *Br Med J* 1995; **310**: 480–481.

[3] Murphy E, Mattson B. Qualitative research and family practice: A marriage made in heaven? *Fam Pract* 1992; **9**: 85–91.

[4] Dowell J, Huby G, Smith C. *Scottish consensus statement on qualitative research in primary care.* 1995: pp. 1–88.

[5] Hamberg K, Johansson E, Lindgren G, Westman G. Scientific rigour in qualitative research-examples from a study of women's health in family practice. *Fam Pract* 1994; **11**: 176–181.

[6] Kai J. Parents' difficulties and information needs in coping with acute illness in pre-school children: a qualitative study. *Br Med J* 1996; **313**: 987–990.

[7] Kai J. What worries parents when their pre-school children are acutely ill, and why: a qualitative study. *Br Med J* 1996; **313**: 983–986.

[8] Dicker A, Armstrong D. Patients' views of priority setting in health care: an interview survey in one practice. *Br Med J* 1995; **311**: 1137–1139.

[9] Kai J. Parents' perceptions of taking babies' rectal temperature. *Br Med J* 1993; **307**: 660–662.

[10] Hopton J, Hogg R, McKee I. Patients' accounts of calling the doctor out of hours: a qualitative study in one general practice. *Br Med J* 1996; **313**: 991–994.

[11] Benson J, Britten N. Respecting the autonomy of cancer patients when talking with their families: qualitative analysis of semistructured interviews with patients. *Br Med J* 1996; **313**: 729–731.

[12] Britten N. Patients' ideas about medicines: a qualitative study in a general practice population. *Br J Gen Pract* 1994; **44**: 465–468.

[13] Mellor J, Chambers N. Addressing the patient's agenda in the reorganisation of ante-natal and infant health care: experience in one general practice. *Br J Gen Pract* 1995; **45**: 423–425.

[14] Carman D, Britten N. Confidentiality of medical records: the patient's perspective. *Br J Gen Pract* 1995; **45**: 485–488.

[15] Skelton AM, Murphy EA, Murphy RJL, O'Dowd TC. Patients' views of low back pain and its management in general practice. *Br J Gen Pract* 1996; **46**: 153–156.

[16] Lewis JR, Williamson V. Examining patient perceptions of quality care in general practice: comparison of quantitative and qualitative methods. *Br J Gen Pract* 1995; **45**: 249–253.

[17] Jones RVH, Greenwood B. Breast cancer: causes of patients distress identified by qualitative analysis. *Br J Gen Pract* 1994; **44**: 370–371.

[18] Ridsdale L, Hudd S. Computers in the consultation: the patient's view. *Br J Gen Pract* 1994; **44**: 367–369.

[19] Cunningham-Burley S, Allbutt H, Garraway WM, Lee AJ, Russell EBAW. Perceptions of urinary symptoms and health care-seeking behaviour amongst men aged 40–79 years. *Br J Gen Pract* 1996; **46**: 349–352.

[20] Fisher B, Britten N. Patient access to records: expectations of hospital doctors and experiences of cancer patients. *Br J Gen Pract* 1993; **43**: 52–56.

[21] Murphy E, Kinmonth AL, Marteau T. General practice based diabetes surveillance: the views of patients. *Br J Gen Pract* 1992; **42**: 279–283.

[22] Cromarty IJ. What do patients think about during their consultations? A qualitative study. *Br J Gen Pract* 1996; **46**: 525–528.

[23] Kai J. Baby check in the inner city – use and value to parents. *Fam Pract* 1994; **11**: 245–249.

[24] Borkan J, Shvartzman P, Reis S, Morris AG. Stories from the sealed rooms: patient interviews during the gulf war. *Fam Pract* 1993; **10**: 188–192.

[25] Cornford CS, Morgan M, Ridsdale L. Why do mothers consult when their children cough? *Fam Pract* 1993; **10**: 193–186.

[26] Brorsson A, Rastam L. The patient's family history: a key to the physician's understanding of patients' fears. *Fam Pract* 1993; **10**: 197–200.

[27] Britten N. Patient demand for prescriptions: a view from the other side. *Fam Pract* 1994; **11**: 62–65.

[28] Murphy E, Kinmonth AL. No symptoms, no problem? Patients' understanding of non-insulin dependent diabetes. *Fam Pract* 1995; **12**: 184–192.

[29] Brorsson A, Troein M, Lindbladh E, Selander S, Widlund M, Rastam L. My family dies from heart attacks. How hypercholesterolaemic men refer to their family history. *Fam Pract* 1995; **12**: 433–437.

[30] Whittaker A. Qualitative methods in general practice research: experience from the Oceanpoint study. *Fam Pract* 1996; **13**: 310–316.

[31] Murray J, Shepherd S. Alternative or additional medicine? An exploratory study in general practice. *Soc Sci Med* 1993; **37**: 983–988.

[32] Borkan J, Reis S, Hermoni D, Biderman A. Talking about the pain: a patient-centred study of low back pain in primary care. *Soc Sci Med* 1995; **40**: 977–988.

[33] Punamaki RL, Kokko SJ. Content and predictors of consultation experiences among Finnish primary care patients. *Soc Sci Med* 1995; **40**: 231–243.

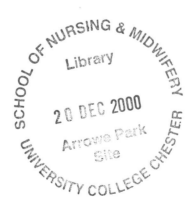